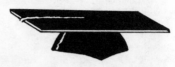

How the Student with Hearing Loss Can Succeed in College: A Handbook for Students, Families and Professionals

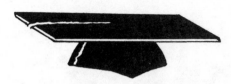

How the Student with Hearing Loss Can Succeed in College: A Handbook for Students, Families and Professionals

Carol Flexer, Ph.D.,
Denise Wray, Ph.D.,
Ron Leavitt, M.S., Editors

Foreword

Mark Ross, Ph.D.

Alexander Graham Bell Association for the Deaf, Inc.
3417 Volta Place, N.W., Washington, D.C. 20007-2778

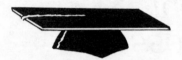

Library of Congress Cataloging in Publication Data

Flexer, Carol, Ph.D., Denise Wray, Ph.D., Ron Leavitt, M.S., Editors
How the Student with a Hearing Loss Can Succeed in College:
A Handbook for Students, Families and Professionals

Library of Congress catalog card number 90-081332
ISBN 0-88200-170-1
© 1990 Alexander Graham Bell Association for the Deaf
3417 Volta Place, N.W.
Washington, D.C. 20007

Printed in the United States of America
10   9   8   7   6   5   4   3   2   1

Dedication

This book is dedicated to college students with hearing loss, and to a future of options and opportunity.

Acknowledgements

This book has evolved with the caring assistance of many people. The editors wish to acknowledge the invaluable help and support of numerous colleagues, family members, and friends; especially faculty and staff of The Department of Communicative Disorders at The University of Akron. Thanks to Kim McCarthy, Julie Scott, and Janeane Brainard for their tireless typing; to Jackie Rios for her art work and Dave Shoenfelt for the photographs; to Pete Flexer and John Wray for their patient support; and to Lucy Cuzon du Rest, Consulting Publications Director at the Alexander Graham Bell Association for the Deaf, and Donald McGee, Alexander Graham Bell Publications Committee Chairman who provided guidance, encouragement and assistance with the manuscript.

Contents

PART III COUNSELING 147

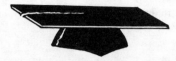

Contributing Authors

Frederick S. Berg, Ph.D.
Professor
Department of Communicative Disorders
Utah State University
Logan, Utah
(Chapter 5)

Thomas S. Black, M.S.
Educational Audiologist
Special Education Regional Resource Center
Hillsboro, Ohio
(Chapter 13)

James C. Blair, Ph.D.
Professor
Department of Communicative Disorders
Utah State University
Logan, Utah
(Chapter 6)

Carol Flexer, Ph.D.
Associate Professor
Department of Communicative Disorders
The University of Akron
Akron, Ohio
(Chapters 1,2,5,13)

John Freeburg, M.A.
Director of the Resource Center for Deafness
Western Oregon State College
Monmouth, Oregon
(Chapter 14)

William R. Hodgson, Ph.D.
Professor
Department of Speech and Hearing Sciences
University of Arizona
Tucson, Arizona
(Chapter 3)

Mary King, M.A.
Coordinator of the Writing Lab
Department of Developmental Programs
The University of Akron
Akron, Ohio
(Chapter 9)

George Kosovich, M.A., M.Ed.
The Northern Regional Coordinator for the
Oregon State Deaf and Hearing-Impaired
Access Program
Portland, Oregon
(Chapter 7)

Ron Leavitt, M.S.
Communication Specialist and Supervisor in
Aural Habilitation
Department of Speech Communication
Oregon State University
Corvallis, Oregon
(Chapters 1,4,12)

Winifred Northcott, Ph.D.
Consultant Lecturer
Oral Interpreting
Minneapolis, Minnesota
(Chapter 11)

Grace E. Olmstead, M.Ed.
Director
Student Services for the Handicapped
The University of Akron
Akron, Ohio
(Chapter 8)

Mark Ross, Ph.D.
Director of Research and Training
New York League for the Hard-of-Hearing
Adjunct Professor of City
University of New York
(Foreword)

Joseph Sendelbaugh, Ed.D.
Associate Professor
Rehabilitation Counseling-Deafness Program
Western Oregon State College
Monmouth, Oregon
(Chapter 14)

Denise Wray, Ph.D.
Associate Professor
Department of Communicative Disorders
The University of Akron
Akron, Ohio
(Chapters 1,10,13)

Student Authors: (Chapter 15)
Susan Coler—The University of Akron
Steve Gordon—The University of Akron
Kathryn Louden—The University of Akron
Doreen McSorley—Western Oregon State College
Peter Paulson—The University of Minnesota
Jenny Schwartzberg—Princeton University
Crystal Terrell—The University of Akron
David Viers—Western Oregon State College
Kim Woods—Western Oregon State College

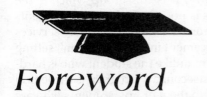

Foreword

Years ago (1977) I wrote a chapter for a monograph which was entitled "Our forgotten children: Hard-of-hearing pupils in the schools." This current book is a reminder that the children of that era, now grown, may still be forgotten and overlooked. From their own experience, Flexer, Wray, and Leavitt document how little the college students with hearing loss with whom they worked understood the ramifications of their own hearing conditions, how poorly they have been fit with amplification and other assistive devices, and how pervasive were their social and communicative problems. The young adults described in this book graduated, for the most part, from mainstream programs and received what must have been considered adequate services for their condition. It is really quite disheartening to contemplate the gap between the services we know to be necessary and what is, apparently, common practice. Organized programs for postsecondary students who are hard-of-hearing cannot only help them, as this book amply demonstrates, but can also illuminate the inadequacy of the support services in their elementary and secondary programs. One can but hope that the current generation of young children with hearing loss will not be so "forgotten" and will enter college better prepared than their older predecessors. We should not have to wait until a person who is hard-of-hearing starts college to realize the insufficiency of their earlier training. How many never get to that point at all, discouraged by poor achievements and poor self-images?

The needs of the average college student who is hard-of-hearing will *not* be met by enrolling him or her in one of the 145 postsecondary programs specifically designed for students who are "deaf" (DeCaro, Karchmer, & Rawlings, 1987). There is a large conceptual and functional difference between individuals who are hard-of-hearing, those whose primary communication mode is auditorially-based, and people who are deaf, whose primary mode of communication is visually-based. There are many more of the former, people with mild, moderate, and severe hearing losses, than there are of the latter, those with profound hearing impairments. Given the demography of hearing impairment, it is probable that there are some students who are hard-of-hearing in every postsecondary institution in the country. It is this group which is the main focus of this book, although this is not to say that some students who are "deaf" cannot also benefit from the kind of support services envisioned here. It is just that their placement in a "mainstream" setting requires a sensitive and explicit decision, unlike the student who is hard-of-hearing for whom a mainstream postsecondary program is the logical choice. In other words, whether we help them or not, students who are hard-of-hearing are still going to be there. As far as I know, the program at The University of Akron is the only one which has specifically targeted young adults for *comprehensive* therapeutic assistance.

The authors have used their experience both to write and to select contributors to this book, the only one which directly addresses the needs of college students who are hard-of-hearing. The editors have called on the talents of a host of professionals, some well known to speech-language pathologists and audiologists, and others with expertise in vocational rehabilitation, academic tutoring of all types, and career counseling. It is a refreshing experience for a rehabilitative oriented audiologist like myself to read about the significant contribution to academic success and social adjustments which can be made to the college student who is hard-of-hearing by our colleagues in other professions. The material is an antidote to professional insularity; what is stressed is the mutual and co-equal effort of a number of specialists, with the students playing a key role in their own rehabilitation.

There is an underlying premise to this book that I couldn't agree with more, and that is that the hearing impairment should not be an insuperable barrier to a successful college experience, in all respects, socially and academically. To date, our professional focus has been on the preschool and elementary-aged child; the successful "rehabilitation" of a person with hearing loss, however, does not terminate automatically at any age. What we have to respond to is need and not age. If we have provided the necessary services early on, then the later needs should be less, but in some respect or other, may still be necessary. For example, many college students who are hard-of-hearing have never met another young person with a comparable problem and most have never experienced the invaluable mutual support offered by periodic group meetings with other young adults with hearing loss. It is at this age that the students are sufficiently mature to understand the implications of their own impairment and attempt to come to terms with what is going to be a life-long condition for them. The hearing loss will not be going away. So the college experience for these young adults, much more than for a college student with normal hearing, is, or should be, a training ground for their future which transcends the purely academic component.

It is, I suppose, not fashionable to think that children who are hard-of-hearing may require an extended therapeutic effort, extending through college and perhaps beyond. Those of us who work with individuals with hearing loss understand the pervasive impact of a hearing loss, an impact not typically understood by the lay public. For many people, the provision of a hearing aid is synonymous with habilitation. The effect of a congenital hearing loss upon speech, language, academics, and psychosocial behavior is imperfectly understood, particularly concerning hard-of-hearing people who can communicate adequately in many situations. We get impatient with inconsistencies and ambiguities, hallmarks in the behavior and performance of most people who are hard-of-hearing. It is difficult for lay people to realize just how tenuous, in many situations, speech comprehension is for many individuals with hearing loss. Noise and reverberation levels which have little effect upon a normal hearing person may make comprehension impossible for a person who is hard-of-hearing. A professor with a heavy accent, whom normal hearing classmates have some, but acceptable difficulty understanding, may be actually talking a different language as far as the student who is hard-of-hearing is concerned. Unfamiliar expressions, difficult syntactic constructions, free-wheeling classroom discussions, important social and extracurricular interactions, may all present inordinate difficulty for the average student who is hard-of-hearing.

Given all these factors, one may well ask, is it all worth it? Why not simply enroll such students in less challenging postsecondary programs, or in one of the programs specifically designed for the "deaf?" This would be an unfortunate conclusion to draw. First, since these students exhibit the same range of basic intellectual capacities as their normal hearing peers, they should be given the same opportunity to use their innate capabilities. Secondly, as I have already mentioned, these students can use the auditory channel as a primary channel for receiving information. (We should understand that reading, an indispensable skill in higher education, is nonetheless grounded on the basic language capacities normally developed through audition.) Technological assistance can enable such students to use their hearing more effectively, coupled with the kind of back-up tutorial assistance contemplated in the following chapters.

This book presents a clinical challenge to those of us who work in training programs for Speech-Language Pathologists and Audiologists. We're committed to training professionals to work with people who are hard-of-hearing; our students work with such clients on an out-patient basis in all of our clinics; we send students out to cooperating institutions for practicum experience; and we often organize aural rehabilitation groups for older adults with hearing losses. Let's look a little closer to home for clients who need and can benefit greatly from our services; that is, the general population of students in our institutions. Students who are hard-of-hearing may not be registered with the Office of Special Student Services, since, as they are not "deaf," they may think that this office has nothing to do with them. They also may not be fully cognizant or accepting of their own condition and what can be done to help them. But they are there, as I personally have often learned. Students who are hard-of-hearing have to be sought out, evaluated, and convinced that there is nothing shameful in seeking appropriate therapeutic assistance. But such assistance, to be fully effective, has to be comprehensive and include the full range of services outlined in this book. I would, of course, extend this challenge to any postsecondary institution. We should serve as an example to all institutions of higher learning. And this book, the first of its type, could well serve as the "bible" for our endeavors.

References

DeCaro, J.J., Karchmer, M.A., & Rawlings, B.W. (1987). Postsecondary programs for deaf students at the peak of the Rubella bulge. *American Annals of the Deaf, 132,* 36–42.

Mark Ross, Ph.D.
Director of Research and Training
New York League for the Hard-of-Hearing
Adjunct Professor of City University of New York

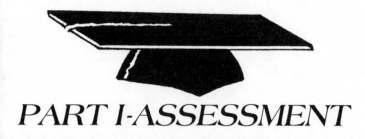

PART I-ASSESSMENT

In a logical manner, this book begins by defining the problem. Chapter 1 profiles college students with hearing loss. Who are they? Where do they come from? How well prepared are they to compete in a hearing university? Chapter 1 raises and then proposes some answers to these questions.

As Mark Ross has said many times, "The problem with having a hearing loss is that you don't hear so good." Thus, Chapter 2 focuses on the core issue of hearing; what exactly is hearing loss, how is hearing tested, and how can the results of a thorough hearing test be meaningfully interpreted?

The most direct way to access residual or remaining hearing is through hearing aids. Chapter 3 focuses on the importance of obtaining an appropriate hearing aid. Where can one get hearing aids? What exactly is a hearing aid evaluation? How can one tell if the hearing aid dispenser really knows what he/she is doing?

Thus, this book "begins at the beginning" by identifying, in a no-nonsense way, the students, their hearing losses, and their hearing aids. The step-by-step chapter format presents technical information in a practical, logical manner.

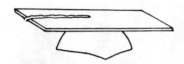

Chapter 1
Overview: The College Student with Hearing Loss

Carol Flexer, Ph.D., Denise Wray, Ph.D., Ron Leavitt, M.S.

For over forty years, rehabilitation information has been provided to professionals who work with students who experience hearing loss on the assumption that these professionals could best educate people with hearing loss and their associates. However, it has often been shown that people with hearing loss do not themselves understand their hearing losses (Flexer, Wray & Black, 1986) and are not familiar with hearing aids and other technology for people with hearing loss (Cranmer, 1985, 1986; Flexer, Wray, & Black, 1986). Further, hearing rehabilitation professionals are not using or promoting available technology for people with hearing loss, and do not seem to be dealing with the important academic, counseling and vocational placement issues of the student with hearing loss (Flexer, Wray, & Black, 1986; Leavitt, 1985, 1987).

This book has been written to promote a better understanding of the needs and possibilities for students who experience hearing loss. It is intended to be used by college students with all degrees of hearing loss from mild to profound, and those who are responsible for their education and habilitation. The underlying philosophy of this book is that with appropriate education, testing, and emotional support, students with hearing loss can become their own best advocates and can participate in their rehabilitation programs. This client-centered orientation does not reduce the important role played by other rehabilitation professionals such as audiologists, speech-language pathologists, classroom teachers, high-school guidance counselors, vocational rehabilitation counselors, special student service personnel, and academic tutors.

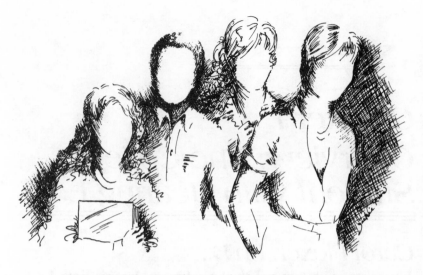

Figure 1-1: Who Are These Beginning College Students?

Indeed, these professionals play a key role in the education, testing, rehabilitation, and counseling of the student with hearing loss. The unusual focus of this book, however, is to place the college student with hearing loss on this team in an important decision making role.

This interdisciplinary text is written by professionals in pivotal positions of the rehabilitation system who have had a great deal of experience with college students who are hearing impaired. Because the book is also intended for the consumer (parents and students), it is written in a style readily understood by both professionals and lay persons. To make it easier for consumer use, a glossary is included at the end of the book, as well as a summary checklist at the end of each chapter. The book is organized into three sections: Assessment, Rehabilitation, and Counseling Issues, highlighting the major areas that must be considered for every college student regardless of the severity of his or her hearing loss.

Profile of Beginning College Students with Hearing Loss

Who are these beginning college students? Where have they been coming from? What are they like? What are the problems which might make it hard for them to adjust to college? It is through understanding their background and needs that we can provide the best services and maximize the potential for success.

1. Type of High School Education:

The students that we have seen have primarily been mainstreamed into regular classrooms during their school years with little or no resource services at the high-school level (Ross, Brackett, & Maxon, 1982). Lack of resource help is not surprising, given that less than one percent of children with hearing loss are being served by our nation's schools (Berg, 1986). Specifically, approximately eight million of the 39.5 million school children have some degree of hearing loss, but only 41,000 students who are hard-of-hearing and 41,000 students who are deaf are actually receiving any kind of special help in schools. Speech-language therapy has often been the service provided for the longest period of time.

2. Type of Communication Skills:

The vast majority have been verbal language users with good intelligibility. They consider themselves to be part of the hearing world. That is, they consider themselves to be persons who are hard-of-hearing, rather than persons who are deaf. Most of their friends are normally hearing.

3. Degree of Hearing Loss:

Consistent with national statistics that over 92 percent of the twenty million persons with hearing loss in this country are functionally hard-of-hearing rather than deaf, most of the students have mild to severe hearing losses (Diedrichsen, 1987). A few have a severe loss in one ear and profound loss in the other. Most have had their hearing losses since birth.

4. Hearing Aids:

All were under-amplified (Flexer & Wray, 1984). That is, their hearing aids were not fit so that they could hear everything that they were capable of hearing. In fact, the majority of the students had unilateral fittings for bilateral hearing losses. Further, amplification was initiated at a late time in terms of speech, language, and auditory development (i.e., some did not wear hearing aids until first or second grade). Their hearing aids did not have strong telecoils and thus could not be attached to Assistive Listening Devices. The bottom line is, all were made to function with unnecessary handicaps due to "less than the best" or even "less than adequate" hearing aid fittings.

5. Students' Knowledge of Their Own Hearing Loss and Hearing Aids:

The vast majority of the college students could not show an understanding of their own type and degree of hearing loss, either unaided or aided (Flexer, Wray, & Black, 1986). They did not understand their hearing aids enough to perform even basic trouble-shooting techniques. They had never used and did not know about Assistive Listening Devices (ALD), including FM systems (an integral part of university life) and telephone amplifiers. This lack of knowledge was not due to low intelligence, but rather due to lack of information. Because of this lack of information, the students were not knowledgeable consumers and so continued to function with unnecessary barriers. Interestingly, there are only 600–700 audiologists in the 16,000 U.S. school districts (Berg, 1986). No wonder these students weren't appropriately advised within a school setting.

6. Use of Services Provided by Federal and State Programs of Vocational Rehabilitation:

The majority of students were eligible for some degree of funding, but did not know that they were. This funding applied to the purchasing of hearing aids for career training. Further, they did not know how to begin to apply for money to help them through college.

7. Preparation for University Coursework:

The majority of students with hearing loss were neither ready nor prepared for university-level coursework as shown by the fact that most needed to take basic skills (remedial) courses in English, reading, writing, and math (Flexer, Wray, & Black, 1986). The students were placed in these courses because of their poor scores on college entrance exams. Most were surprised by this turn of events. In addition, most students could not handle a full course load due to problems with reading and writing.

8. Language Skills:

Most of the students had difficulty with secondary language skills such as reading, writing, and vocabulary comprehension and use, as shown by scores on several language tests. These are subtle language difficulties that may not have been obvious in high school but nonetheless, negatively impacted on academic performance.

9. Knowledge of the Services Available to Them at the University:

Most students did not know that they qualified for special help from the university. The university's Department of Handicapped Student Services helps students deal with other departments in the university. Ironically, many students said that if they took advantage of these services (e.g., scheduling preferences, ALD's provided, tutoring, speech/language/hearing services, extended test-taking time, etc.) they felt as if they were cheating, even though they were entitled to and truly needed these services in order to do well in college.

10. Attitude:

Many students with hearing loss did not have a special group of friends in college and reported feeling quite lonely. Therefore, a support-information group was developed to help deal with emotional and educational needs. Many students came to the university still feeling ashamed of their hearing loss, embarrassed to have classmates "know," and hesitant to tell teachers. Many stated that they would rather flunk a course than tell the teacher that they have a hearing loss and might need some special help.

11. Knowledge of Legal Rights:

Most of the students had no idea of their legal rights as persons who are hearing impaired, in both school and job situations.

12. Knowledge of Career Choices:

Most of the students had no idea how their hearing losses could or could not affect them in certain careers. Therefore, career choices were hastily or unrealistically made, or often unnecessarily dismissed.

13. Academic Help Available:

Many students had been afraid to go to a "hearing" college because they had trouble with school work. However, most universities, especially those with a policy of open enrollment, have a Developmental Program Department. These departments provide the help necessary for a student to compete in college courses.

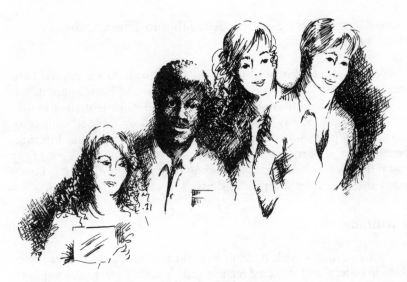

Figure 1-2: Appropriate Information and Support Services Could Facilitate Success in College.

The bottom line is, most students with hearing loss, like other freshmen, entered the university in a very helpless state, but one which was compounded by a hearing loss. They did not know what to expect from university work. Most important, they did not understand how their hearing losses could affect them in college, and thus, could not begin to ask for help. They continued to be victimized by their hearing losses, and not to know how to solve the problem. The results of this lack of knowledge could cause them to fail out of school, to make the wrong career choices, and to experience a lonely existence in college. The saddest thing that could happen is that these students could experience failure during what could possibly be the most important time of their lives. **All of this may be unnecessary, given information and support.**

Checklist for a Successful, Cohesive Service-Delivery System at the College Level

1. **Good audiological services,** including an educational audiologist who is able to explain the impact of the student's hearing loss on communicative and educational function (Chapter 2).

2. **State-of-the-art amplification** to access all residual hearing (Chapters 3 & 4).

3. Accessibility of appropriate **Assistive Communication Devices** (Chapters 5 & 6).

4. Availability of **funding sources** (Chapter 7).

5. A university department of **Special Student Services** to advise students of supportive services and accommodations to which they are entitled (Chapters 8 & 11).

6. A university **Department of Developmental Programming** (basic skills or preparatory classes) to manage existing academic deficits; specifically in math, reading, English, and writing (Chapter 9).

7. Availability of **speech-language services** (Chapter 10).

8. Understanding and **acceptance of hearing loss** (Chapter 12).

9. A peer **support group** (Chapters 12, 13, & 15).

10. Advice about **career options** (Chapter 14).

References

Berg, F.S. (1986). Characteristics of the target population (pp. 1–24). In F.S. Berg, J.C. Blair, S.H. Viehweg, & A. Wilson-Vlotman (Eds.), *Educational Audiology for the Hard-of-Hearing Child*. Orlando, FL: Grune & Stratton.

Cranmer, K.S. (1985). Hearing aid dispensing 1985. *Hearing Instruments, 36*, 6.

Cranmer, K.S. (1986). Hearing aid dispensing 1986. *Hearing Instruments, 37*, 8.

Diedrichsen, R. (1987). Towards the acquisition of basic rights and services for persons who are hard of hearing. *SHHH, 8*, 3–4.

Flexer, C. & Wray, D. (1984). Congenitally hearing impaired college students: The forgotten group. *Hearing Instruments, 35*, 20; 49.

Flexer, C., Wray, D.F., & Black, T.S. (1986). Support group for moderately hearing impaired college students: An expanding awareness. *The Volta Review, 88*, 223–229.

Leavitt, R.J. (1985). Counseling to encourage use of SNR enhancing systems. *Hearing Instruments, 36*, 8–9.

Leavitt, R.J. (1987). Promoting the use of rehabilitation technology. *ASHA, 29*, 28–31.

Ross, M., Brackett, D., & Maxon, A. (1982). *Hard-of-Hearing Children in Regular Schools*. Englewood Cliffs, NJ: Prentice Hall, Inc.

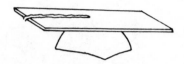

Chapter 2
Hearing for Success: The Importance of Understanding and Measuring Hearing Loss

Carol Flexer, Ph.D.

The authors of this book have found that the majority of college students across the country do not know very much about their hearing losses (Flexer & Wray, 1984; Flexer, Wray, & Black, 1986). That is, the students could not explain the type and degree of their hearing losses, nor did they have an understanding about how and why their hearing losses interfered with communication. It certainly does not make sense to have a hearing test unless results of that test are meaningful. So, this chapter will discuss how hearing fits into one's life, how the ear works, how the ear breaks down, and how to measure hearing loss.

What Is Hearing Loss?

Because one cannot "see" the hearing loss, it's easy to believe that the loss really doesn't matter too much. In fact, hearing loss acts like an invisible acoustic filter that interferes with incoming sounds (Ling, 1989). To explain, hearing loss is not a mere loss of loudness. Rather, sounds are often "smeared" together, causing them to be distorted. Speech, therefore, might be **audible**, but not **intelligible**. A person with a hearing loss might hear other people speaking, but not be able to hear one speech sound as distinct from another. Words like *invitation* and *vacation* might sound the same, and words like *ladder*, *leader*, *little* and *walk*, *walked*, and

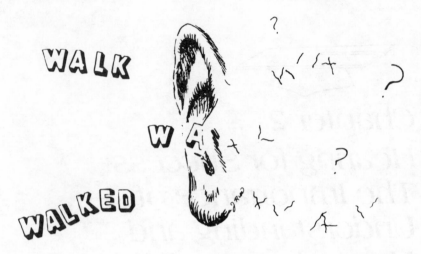

Figure 2-1: Hearing Loss Acts Like an Invisible Acoustic Filter That Interferes with Incoming Sounds.

walks could be impossible to distinguish individually. It's not difficult to imagine what such word confusions could do to a child's vocabulary and conceptual language development.

This "acoustic filter" effect is the beginning, the cause, of a whole chain of negative events (Figure 2-1). If sounds, especially speech sounds, are not heard clearly, then one cannot speak clearly. The second step in this chain involves reading ability. If one does not have good speech and language skills, then reading will also suffer. Said another way, we speak because we hear, and we read because we speak. Certainly then, if reading skills are below average, the individual will probably have problems doing well in school. Therefore, since hearing loss is the **cause** of speech/language, reading, and academic difficulties, it makes sense to deal directly with that hearing loss. It is vital to measure that loss accurately, to reach all possible residual hearing (via amplification and assistive listening devices), and to understand truly the nature of that hearing loss (Ross, 1981; Ross & Calvert, 1984).

How Does Hearing Fit into Our Lives

Hearing plays an important role in many aspects of our lives. Some of the purposes of hearing are not obvious. It is often helpful to think of the functions of hearing occurring on three levels: primitive, signal warning, and symbolic (Davis, & Silverman, 1978).

The primitive level is the most hidden, the one of which we are least aware. This level carries the **auditory background**, those sounds which help to identify a location. For example, a school has different sounds than an office building, which sounds different from a grocery store. If a place does not sound as we expect it to sound, we often become very nervous.

We also hear our own biological sounds at this primitive level. We may hear ourselves breathing, or our hearts beating, or our own chewing. A new hearing aid might, because it amplifies sounds differently than the old aid, change the auditory background. This change could make the wearer anxious and nervous without knowing why. Getting used to a new auditory background could be one reason why it might take at least one month to adjust to a new hearing aid, or to a new assistive listening device.

The second and more obvious level of hearing, **signal warning**, has to do with monitoring the environment. Hearing is called a distance sense because it allows us to know what is happening away from our bodies. We don't have to see to know what is going on. For example, a person could be sitting in a dark room, and hear cars, skateboards, typewriters, people talking, and dogs barking. We feel secure when we know what is happening around us, and we often feel anxious when we don't know. Unfortunately, people with hearing losses (even when wearing aids) have a reduced ability to hear accurately over distances; the greater the hearing loss, the greater the reduction in distance hearing or "earshot." That is why we need to speak closer to a person with a hearing loss, and to actively teach speech and language skills to a child who is born with a hearing loss, even a mild to moderate loss.

A person with a hearing loss cannot "overhear" what people are saying, or the events that are occurring. Persons with hearing losses need to pay active attention or information will not be learned. If their attention drifts and they daydream for even a moment, then they are lost. So, this monitoring function of hearing, this ability to hear over distances is crucial for learning and for peace of mind. Persons with hearing losses need to know their range or **distance of hearing**, how far they can *accurately* hear (it could be two inches or two yards). If that range is limited, then the person who is hearing impaired needs to compensate by changing the environment, e.g., move closer to the speaker and remove background sounds, or use assistive listening devices (Flexer, Wray & Ireland, 1989; Leavitt, 1987; Sudler & Flexer, 1986; Zelski & Zelski, 1985).

The third level of hearing, **symbolic**, is the most obvious level. In fact, it was discussed under the previous section, "What Is Hearing Loss?" Speech develops naturally because we hear. If one does not hear well, then speech does not develop well or naturally. That is, speech and language skills often must be actively taught to someone with a hearing loss.

How Is the Ear Put Together?

The human ear is an incredible mechanism. Because the ear does not look very impressive, it is often difficult to appreciate its complexity. For example, our range of sensitivity to sound, from the softest sound that we can just barely hear to a sound loud enough to cause discomfort, is 10,000,000 to 1 (Martin, 1986). The normal ear is so sensitive that it can detect a pressure change equal to 1/5000th of 1/8 of a postage stamp. Animal hearing is not more sensitive than ours in terms of loud/soft sounds. Rather, animals often have different frequency or pitch ranges. Human frequency range is from 20–20,000 Hz (cycles per second). Dogs can hear up to 35,000 Hz, mice up to 65,000 Hz and porpoises up to 135,000 Hz. This difference in frequency or pitch range is what allows some animals to hear sounds, like a dog whistle, that are not audible to humans.

Most of the structure of the human ear is inside the head. The only part that is visible is the pinna, or outer ear. As noted in Figure 2-2, the ear can actually be divided into several portions; the conductive portion or mechanism, the sensorineural mechanism, and the central mechanism.

The conductive mechanism is comprised of the **outer ear** (pinna and ear canal), and **middle ear** (ear drum and air-filled space containing the three smallest bones in the body). The purpose of the conductive system is to get the sounds into the sensorineural system as efficiently as possible.

The sensorineural mechanism is composed of the cochlea **(inner ear)** and eighth cranial nerve. The cochlea contains the thousands of very tiny receptors that actually receive the sound, rather as the retina of the eye receives visual signals. The inner ear also contains the vestibular or balance system.

The central portion of the auditory system is housed in the brainstem and cortex. This central system is very complex and contains billions of neurons in multiple patterns of connections.

In summary, the outer, middle, and inner ear are also known as the peripheral system and function together to "receive" sounds. The brainstem and cortex of the central nervous system function to "perceive" or to understand the sounds sent to it from the peripheral system. The purpose of a basic hearing test is to measure the function of the peripheral system in order to determine how well sound is being "re-

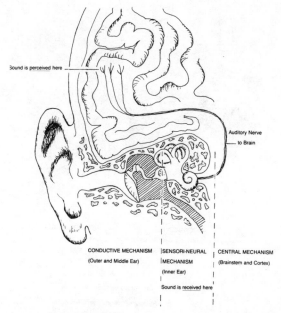

Figure 2-2: The Ear Can Be Divided into the Conductive, the Sensori-neural, and the Central Mechanism.

ceived" (Hodgson, 1980). Hearing aids can help the reception of sound. There are additional tests which can measure perception, a more complex function. Hearing aids do not help perception, rather perception is learned. For example, if an English speaking person with normal hearing visits Japan, he/she probably won't understand or perceive what people are saying. Wearing a hearing aid will not help the English speaking person to understand Japanese any better.

What Happens When the Ear Breaks Down?

Hearing losses happen for a reason. That is, hearing losses are caused by damage or disease somewhere in the auditory system (ear). There are three general categories of hearing loss based upon where in the ear the damage occurs: conductive, sensorineural, and mixed (Northern, 1984). See Figure 2-3.

A **conductive-type hearing loss** means that the "site of lesion," or location of the damage, is in the outer or middle ear. Many conductive hearing losses can be corrected by medical or surgical treatment because the conductive system functions to "conduct" sound and does not contain nerve endings.

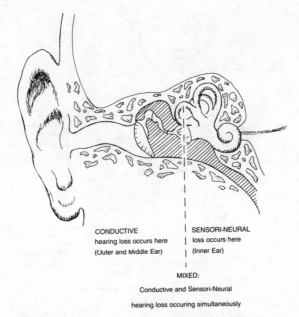

CONDUCTIVE
hearing loss occurs here
(Outer and Middle Ear)

SENSORI-NEURAL
loss occurs here
(Inner Ear)

MIXED:

Conductive and Sensori-Neural

hearing loss occuring simultaneously

Figure 2-3: There Are Three General Categories of Hearing Loss Based Upon Where in the Ear the Damage Occurs: Conductive, Sensori-neural, and Mixed.

The most common conductive hearing loss is otitis media or middle-ear infection. This pathology or disease usually causes a mild to moderate degree of hearing loss (Northern & Downs, 1984) due to fluid collecting in the normally air-filled middle ear space. This fluid may occur with or without active infection, but it *always* causes hearing loss. Infants and young children have the highest incidence of otitis media, which is usually treated with antibiotics. If a person has repeated ear infections and medication does not work, then tiny ventilating tubes may be surgically inserted through the ear drum to allow the middle ear space to remain air-filled.

Hearing aids may be recommended in conjunction with medical treatment for someone with repeated and continual ear infections. That is, both medical and educational management is necessary for someone with repeated bouts of otitis media.

Other examples of conductive-type pathologies include: otosclerosis (stapes footplate fixation), atresia (complete closure of the ear canal), cholesteatoma (a nonmalignant tumor or cyst in the middle ear, often a result of chronic ear infections), mastoiditis (infection of the mastoid process, part of the middle ear structure), stenosis (an abnormally small ear canal), and cerumen impaction (too much ear wax).

A **sensorineural hearing loss** is caused by damage or pathology occurring in the inner ear (cochlea), that part of the ear which contains thousands of tiny receptive nerve endings. Medical treatment cannot repair these nerve endings. Hearing aids and assistive listening devices are typically recommended for sensorineural type losses. Amplification does not "correct" the damage to the inner ear. Rather, amplification functions to shape the incoming sounds to make these sounds easier to hear.

Congenital hearing losses are those which occur before the child has learned speech and language, typically before or at birth (Northern, & Downs, 1984), whereas acquired losses occur after speech and language have been developed. Congenital or acquired losses may be further divided into endogenous (genetic), and exogenous (environmental). Genetic hearing losses are hereditary and have differing probabilities of being passed on to offspring. Exogenous hearing losses, on the other hand, cannot be transmitted to offspring because they are caused by external environmental events, not by the individual's genes. Rubella, cytomegalovirus, bacterial infections (maternal or infant), and anoxia (not enough oxygen before or at birth) are some examples of external agents which could cause a hearing loss.

Other examples of causes of sensorineural hearing loss include: Presbycusis (hearing loss due to aging); noise-induced hearing loss (repeated exposure to loud sounds); ototoxicity (a "poisoning" of the inner ear by high doses of some medications such as mycin drugs, some diuretics, quinine, and aspirin); perilymphatic fistula (a leak in the oval or round window, both being points of communication between the middle and inner ear); acoustic neuroma, also called an eighth nerve tumor (a nonmalignant tumor which grows off of the main nerve trunk that carries auditory sensations from the inner ear to the brain . . . a brainstem tumor which causes hearing loss, and could be fatal if not diagnosed and surgically removed); and Ménière's disease (excessive fluid pressure in the *inner* ear which can cause dizziness, hearing loss, and tinnitus). **Tinnitus** is a ringing, buzzing, or chirping sound inside one's head, and it often accompanies sensorineural hearing loss. This ringing can be constant or infrequent, and range from barely noticeable to terribly destructive. For more detailed discussions of ear pathologies, the reader is referred to Martin (1986), and to Northern (1984).

A mixed hearing loss means that the person has several pathologies existing at the same time causing *both* conductive and sensorineural hearing losses. For example, an individual might have otitis media (ear infection) on top of a congenital sensorineural hearing loss. Both hearing losses would need to be identified and managed. Once the hearing losses are identified by an audiologist, a physician diagnoses the specific pathologies which are the cause of the hearing losses. The physician can then medically manage, through medication or surgery, those hearing losses which can be medically treated (mostly conductive-type hearing losses). The **audiologist provides nonmedical management of hearing losses**, such as appropriate fitting and use of hearing aids and assistive listening devices, and habilitative treatment in the form of speech and language stimulation, auditory training/learning, and speechreading (Berg, Blair, Viehweg, & Wilson-Vlotman, 1986).

Two other categories of hearing loss should be mentioned at this point: central and functional. A **central hearing loss** is not really a "hearing loss" relative to loss of reception. Rather, a central auditory problem causes difficulty with the perception or understanding of incoming sounds. A stroke, head trauma, or congenital brain damage could cause problems with understanding what is being said even though the sounds are "getting in" just fine. A **functional hearing loss** is not really a hearing loss, either. Rather, the person (adult or child) is faking a hearing loss or exaggerating an existing hearing loss.

How Does Sound Reach Our Ears?

Sound can reach our ears by two pathways, and both are utilized in a hearing test (Martin, 1986). The most efficient and obvious pathway is called **air conduction**. Sound travels through the air from a source (another speaker, for example), reaches our ears and enters the auditory system through the ear canal, progressing through the eardrum, middle ear, inner ear (where sensory receptors and nerve endings are), and up the brainstem to the cortex or brain where perception occurs.

The second and less obvious pathway for hearing is called **bone conduction**. In bone conduction, sound bypasses the conductive system (outer and middle ear), and directly reaches the inner ear. Because the inner ear is deep inside the skull (specifically, inside the temporal bone), anything which causes the head to vibrate could also cause the inner ear to vibrate.

What Happens When a Person Has a Hearing Test?

A basic hearing evaluation is actually comprised of several tests, collectively called a **"test battery."** A test battery approach provides detailed information, avoids drawing conclusions from a single test, and allows for the detection of multiple pathologies (Hannley, 1986). The following tests are contained in a typical test battery: case history, tuning fork tests, speech threshold test, speech discrimination testing (also called word identification), pure tone air conduction testing, pure tone bone conduction testing, immittance testing, and counseling the client about the results.

The testing is conducted by an **audiologist**, a certified and licensed individual with a graduate degree in the assessment and nonmedical management of hearing loss. To insure accurate results, hearing tests are performed in an exceptionally quiet place, called a **"sound room."** Any noise could interfere with a person's ability to hear very soft sounds. In addition, a special piece of equipment, an **audiometer** is used. The audiometer allows all speech and tone signals to be carefully measured and controlled in order to obtain accurate results.

l. Case History

The case history is an important part of a hearing test because information can be obtained about factors which could have caused hearing loss, and about the impact of that loss on the person's life.

2. Tuning Fork Tests

Tuning fork tests, performed in the sound room, can provide a quick, subjective estimate about type and degree of hearing loss (Figure 2-4). Tuning forks have been around for years and are typically used by **otologists** (physicians who are ear specialists), as well as by audiologists.

3. Speech Threshold Test

A Speech Recognition Threshold (also called a Speech Reception Threshold or SRT) is the softest level at which an individual can barely understand speech 50 percent of the time. In fact, anytime the word "threshold" is used, it means that point at which the individual can just barely hear a sound. Spondees, two syllable words, (e.g., baseball, cowboy, hot dog, ice cream, snowman), are the speech materials typically used for this task.

4. Speech Discrimination Testing, Also Called Word Identification Test

Speech discrimination tests are the second of two speech tests typically used in a basic test battery, SRT being the first. Whereas SRT

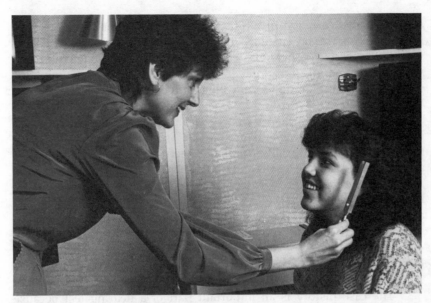

Figure 2-4: Tuning Fork Tests Can Provide a Quick, Subjective Estimate of Type and Degree of Hearing Loss.

is a threshold task, discrimination words are presented at levels louder than threshold. Two questions are typically answered by discrimination testing: a) How well can the client understand speech at an average conversational level of loudness, approximately 45 dB HL? b) How well can the client understand speech when the words are presented loud enough to overcome the hearing loss? It's rather like comparing how well a person can understand words when one uses a normal conversational voice to when one shouts.

5. Pure Tone Air Conduction Testing

This is the hearing test that many people have had at one time or another. Whistle-like sounds are presented through the headphones to each ear separately, and the client raises his/her hand each time the tone is just barely heard (Figure 2-5). The tones vary in frequency or pitch in octave intervals from 250 Hz (approximately middle "C" on the piano) through 8000 Hz. These particular pitches were selected as the test tones because collectively they make up speech sounds, much like individual threads form a cloth (Ling, 1989). One is not consciously aware of the individual pure tones comprising someone's speech anymore than one is aware of each individual thread when one sees a dress.

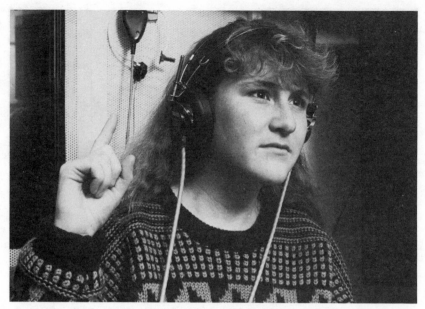

Figure 2-5: For Pure Tone Air Conduction Testing, the Client Wears Headphones, Sits in a Sound Room, and Raises Her Hand Every Time the Whistle-like Sound Is Heard, Even If It Is Very Soft.

Nevertheless, there is a relationship between each pure tone and individual speech sounds. For example, if one can detect (hear) the low frequency (low pitch) pure tones (250 Hz and 500 Hz), then one can hear many vowel sounds and the melody of speech. If one can detect 2000 Hz, then all consonants except s/z will be audible. If one cannot detect 4000 Hz (a very high pitch sound), then one cannot hear the s/z speech sound. Not hearing the /s/ means more than simply not hearing the "snake" sound. For a child who is still learning speech and language, not hearing /s/ means not hearing the concepts of plurality, possessives, first person, etc.

It is important once again to make a distinction between "audibility" and "intelligibility" of speech. Hearing tests help to determine if speech is merely audible (one knows someone is speaking), or if speech is potentially intelligible. Intelligibility means being able to hear the differences among speech sounds; for example, being able to hear the words *manner*, *matter*, and *master* as distinct and separate words. Certainly, understanding the meaning of these words is a perceptual/learning task. However, if the sounds are not "detected" as unique, then perception or learning cannot occur.

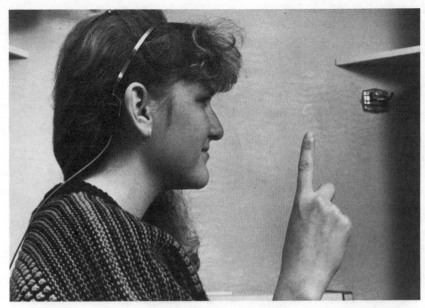

Figure 2-6: Bone Conduction Thresholds Are Obtained with the Client Wearing a Special Piece of Equipment Called a Bone Oscillator.

6. Pure Tone Bone Conduction Testing

As mentioned above, pure tone air conduction testing is performed with the individual wearing headphones. Testing by bone conduction uses a different piece of equipment, called a bone oscillator (Figure 2-6). The bone oscillator is a small, black box attached to a headband which is placed on the head. The signal from the audiometer causes the black box to vibrate, which in turn causes the skull to vibrate, stimulating hearing by bone conduction. That is, in bone conduction testing, the outer and middle ears are bypassed and the inner ear is stimulated directly. Because bone conduction thresholds are obtained by bypassing the conductive mechanism, they can be used to determine **site of lesion** (where in the auditory system the pathology or problem occurs).

During a hearing test, it is not unusual for the audiologist to have to use a masking procedure. **Masking** is the introduction of a specific noise signal, which sounds like static, into the nontest ear through the headphones. The purpose of masking is to make sure that the test ear is in fact the ear that is responding, and that the nontest ear is not contaminating the procedure.

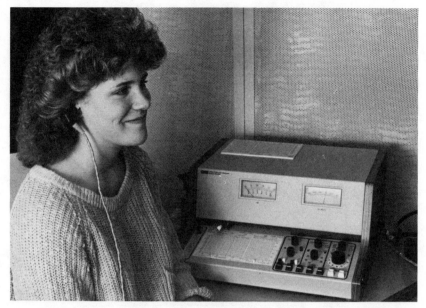

Figure 2-7: For Immittance Testing, the Client Need Only Sit Still and Let the Audiologist and Equipment Do All the Work of Measuring Middle Ear Function.

7. Immittance Testing

The purpose of immittance (also called impedance, or admittance) testing is to obtain an objective measure of middle ear function (pressure, compliance, and mobility). A small, soft rubber probe is inserted in the outside of the ear canal, and a continuous tone is presented accompanied by small air pressure changes which cause the eardrum to move (see Figure 2-7).

8. Counseling the Client about Results of the Hearing Test

One of most important parts of a hearing test is discussing the results in a meaningful way with the client. Finding out about the type and degree of hearing loss is only the first step of an effective hearing test (Hannley, 1986). Exploring the effects of that hearing loss on the client's everyday function is the pivotal second step.

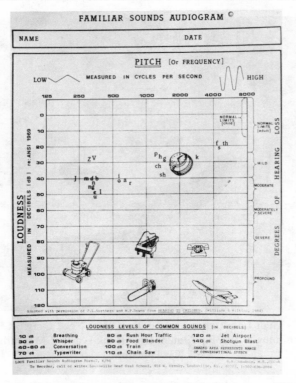

Figure 2-8: This Audiogram Shows Not Only Frequency (Pitch) and Intensity (Loudness), but also the Relationship of Both to Speech and Environmental Sounds.

What Is an Audiogram and What Does It Mean?

An **audiogram** is a simple graph of an individual's hearing sensitivity, which shows type (conductive, sensorineural, mixed), degree (mild-profound), and pattern (how much of a hearing loss exists at the various frequencies) of hearing loss. Frequency (pitch), from 250 Hz through 8000 Hz, is displayed along the top of the graph, and intensity (loudness) in dB (decibels) is shown along the side (Figure 2-8). The higher the number of decibels, the louder the sound. The threshold sensitivity of each ear is displayed individually using the following symbols:

a) 0 = the softest sound the person can hear with his/her right ear under headphones. All sounds louder than threshold (towards the bottom of the graph) would be audible to the person, and sounds softer than threshold (towards the top of the graph), would not.

b) X = the softest sound that the person can hear with his/her left ear under headphones.

c) $\wedge$ = the softest sound that the person can hear when his/her hearing is tested by bone conduction. This symbol does not specify which ear is responding.

All of these symbols specify that the nontest ear was not masked, or removed from the test situation. There are different symbols used when masking is employed, and a legend should be included on every audiogram which defines all symbols used on the graph.

d) S = sound field thresholds. This symbol means that earphones were not used. Rather, the tones were presented through large speakers directly into the sound room. Sound field thresholds are often obtained when a young child won't wear headphones, or when the audiologist wants to compare an individual's aided and unaided thresholds.

What Are Aided Thresholds?

The only way that an individual knows which tones are audible through his or her hearing aid(s) or assistive listening device is to obtain **aided thresholds** (see Chapter 3). That is, one cannot look at an unaided audiogram and "know" which frequencies the person can actually detect while wearing his or her hearing aid(s).

If an assistive listening device is used (e.g., an FM unit worn during school), thresholds should also be obtained when the person is wearing that unit.

Summary

Questions That Should Be Answered by Having a Hearing Test

Following is a **checklist** of questions that should be answered by the audiologist performing a hearing test:

1. Is hearing normal or is there a hearing loss?
2. If hearing loss is present, what type of hearing loss is it (conductive, sensorineural, or mixed)? What degree is the loss (mild to profound)?
3. How can this hearing loss affect communication ability relative to speech intelligibility, distance, and noise?
4. Is the hearing loss stable or is it getting worse?

5. Is it necessary to see an otologist (physician who is an ear specialist) to be examined for potential ear pathology or disease?

6. Have special tests, for example understanding speech in noise, been administered? Since noisy situations are a real problem for persons with hearing loss, it is important to evaluate the specific impact of noise on the individual.

7. Could aural rehabilitation therapy, in the form of auditory training, and/or lipreading be helpful?

8. Could speech/language therapy be helpful? (See Chapter 10.)

9. Are there any support groups available? (See Chapters 13 & 15.)

10. Is the individual's present hearing aid functioning well? Are there any new technological advances that could improve speech intelligibility? (See Chapter 4.) Is a new hearing aid evaluation in order? (See Chapter 3.)

11. Which assistive listening devices could be helpful given the person's lifestyle? (See Chapters 5 & 6.)

12. Could the Vocal Rehabilitation agency provide assistance to the individual? (See Chapter 7.)

13. If the client is a student, are there special educational needs? (See Chapters 8, 9, 11 & 13.)

14. Will a written report and audiogram be mailed to the consumer for home files?

In addition to the above considerations, hearing loss should be monitored at least once a year or more often if changes occur. Note that a **yearly hearing test**, performed by an audiologist, could and should provide educational as well as assessment information.

What to Tell Other People About Your Hearing Loss

Working with college students who experience hearing loss has revealed that many of the students are puzzled about what to tell people about their hearing loss. Chapter 12 will discuss that "Hearing loss is O.K.." The issues in this chapter relate to how to describe hearing loss to others in a way that could facilitate communication. For example, one student stated that a recent acquaintance should have "known" that conversation couldn't be heard in the noisy lunchroom. When asked how the friend should have known, the student replied, "Well, he must have seen my hearing aids." In fact, the hearing aids could not be seen under the student's hair. And even if the aids were visible, how should the friend know about difficult listening situations? The point is, most people would probably be considerate given a chance. But, people need information about hearing loss, and about how hearing loss affects communication.

The following are bits of information which could be helpful in explaining hearing loss to an uninformed person:

1. Compare aided and unaided hearing ability relative to hearing conversational-level speech. For example, "Without my hearing aids, I can just barely hear you talking, but I can't understand anything that you say. That's because, without my aids, I hear low pitch sounds better than high pitch sounds. But, with my aids, I can hear all speech sounds, if the room is relatively quiet and you are close."

2. One could add that the hearing loss is a "nerve" loss (if it's sensorineural), and that the loss has been present since birth (if it is congenital).

3. Perhaps elaborate that noise and distance make understanding difficult.

4. Add that facing the person assists in lipreading, a supplement to hearing.

5. Provide hints of what the person can do if you do not understand him/her. For example, move closer, speak slower (not necessarily louder), rephrase, turn off competing sounds (TV, radio, etc.). (See Chapter 12).

Hearing for Success

Because accessing and utilizing all possible residual hearing is pivotal to academic success, this chapter has focused on understanding and measuring hearing loss. Obtaining thorough and ongoing hearing tests enables one to measure and define the problem. Knowledge of the relationship of one's hearing loss to communication skill, gives one control over the impact of that hearing loss in an academic situation. Indeed, one always must be mindful of the importance of "Hearing for Success."

References

Berg, F.S., Blair, J.C., Viehweg, S.H., & Wilson-Vlotman, A. (1986). *Educational audiology for the hard of hearing child*. Orlando, FL: Grune & Stratton.

Davis, H., & Silverman, S.R. (1978). *Hearing and deafness* (4th ed.). New York: Holt, Rinehart and Winston.

Flexer, C., & Wray, D. (1984). Congenitally hearing impaired college students: The forgotten group. *Hearing Instruments, 35,* 20; 49.

Flexer, C., Wray, D.F., & Black, T.S. (1986). Support group for moderately hearing impaired college students: An expanding awareness. *The Volta Review, 88,* 223–229.

Flexer, C., Wray, D., & Ireland, J. (1989). Preferential seating is not enough: Issues in classroom management of hearing impaired students. *Language, Speech, and Hearing Services in Schools, 20,* 11–21.

Hannley, M. (1986). *Basic principles of auditory assessment.* San Diego, CA: College-Hill Press.

Hodgson, W.R. (1980). *Basic audiologic evaluation.* Baltimore, MD: Williams & Wilkins.

Leavitt, R.J. (1987). Promoting the use of rehabilitation technology. *ASHA, 29,* 28–31.

Ling, D. (1989). *Foundations of spoken language for hearing impaired children.* Washington, DC: The Alexander Graham Bell Association for the Deaf.

Ling, D., & Ling, A.H. (1978). *Aural habilitation the foundations of verbal learning in hearing impaired children.* Washington, DC: The Alexander Graham Bell Association for the Deaf.

Martin, F.N. (1986). *Introduction to audiology* (3rd ed.). Englewood Cliffs, NJ: Prentice-Hall.

Northern, J.L. (Ed.). (1984). *Hearing disorders* (2nd ed.). Boston: Little, Brown and Company.

Northern, J.L. & Downs, M.P. (1984). *Hearing in children* (3rd ed.). Baltimore, MD: Williams & Wilkins.

Ross, M. (1981). Classroom amplification. In W.R. Hodgson & R.H. Skinner (Eds.), *Hearing aid assessment and use in audiologic habilitation* (2nd ed.; pp. 234–257). Baltimore, MD: Williams & Wilkins

Ross, M., & Calvert, D.R. (1984). Semantics of deafness revisited: Total communication and the use and misuse of residual hearing. *Audiology, 9,* 127–145.

Sudler, W.H., & Flexer, C. (1986). Low cost assistive listening device. *Language Speech and Hearing Services in Schools, 17,* 342–344.

Zelski, R.F.K., & Zelski, T. (1985). What are assistive devices? *Hearing Instruments, 36,* 12; 36.

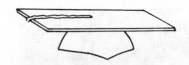

Chapter 3
What to Look For in a Hearing-Aid Evaluation

William R. Hodgson, Ph.D.

Introduction

If you are a college student who is hearing impaired, chances are you have already purchased several hearing aids. In spite of this experience, it is possible that you may not entirely understand the hearing aid selection-recommendation procedure, or know which of several possible procedures is best, and even at that you may not have been buying the best possible amplification for the least possible money. On the other hand, you may be thinking about purchasing your first hearing aids, either because of a recently acquired hearing loss or because the increased demands of college listening cause you to need amplification for the first time. Therefore, whether you are a veteran or a new hearing aid user, I hope the following information will be helpful.

What a Hearing Aid Is (and Isn't)

Even if you have worn hearing aids for a long time, you may not exactly have a handle on their basic nature. Simply stated, a hearing aid is an amplifier. It makes sounds you can't hear audible and in general makes sounds louder. Today's hearing aids perform this function in a very sophisticated way, and avoid many problems present earlier. As shown in Figure 3-1 A and B, the microphone changes sound energy into an electric signal. The amplifier draws power from the battery to enlarge the electric energy. The earphone (receiver) changes the electric signal back into sound energy, so that you can hear it. The earmold holds the aid in the ear and performs other important functions, described later. In Figure 3-2, various hearing aid styles are shown.

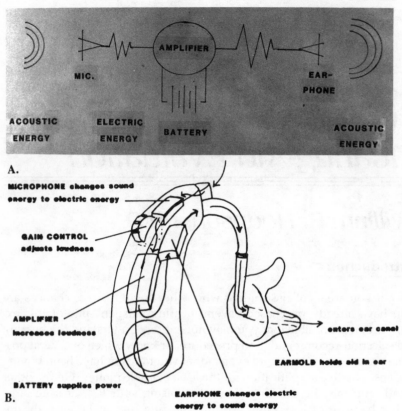

Figure 3-1 A&B: A. Block Diagram of the Amplification Process. The Microphone Turns Acoustic Energy into an Electric Signal, the Amplifier Draws Power from the Battery to Increase that Signal, and the Earphone Turns It Back into Sound Energy.   B. Drawing of a Behind-the-Ear Hearing Aid, Showing Important Parts and Controls.

If you think of a hearing aid as an amplifier, you can see its basic strength and greatest limitation. Today, hearing aids are available with enough power to make at least some sounds audible for people with very severe hearing losses.

The ultimate limitation of the hearing aid amplifier is the condition of your ear. Almost everyone who wears hearing aids has a sensorineural loss. That is, the problem is located in the inner ear or auditory nerve (see Chapter 2). In addition to a loss of hearing sensitivity, disorders of this sort create a loss of speech clarity because of damage to the thousands of sensory cells or nerve fibers which analyze sound waves and send nerve patterns to the brain. If, after the aid makes sounds audible, your ear works well enough to permit you to differentiate sounds, you

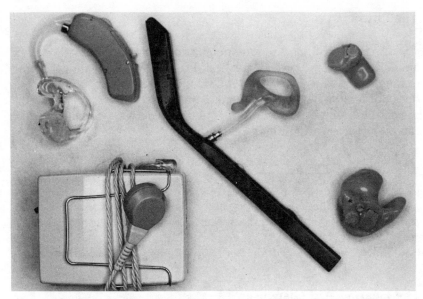

Figure 3-2: Various Hearing-Aid Styles.   A. Body-Worn Aid.   B. Behind-the-Ear Aid.   C. Eyeglass Aid.   D. In-the-Ear Aid.   E. Canal Aid.

will understand amplified speech well. However, the greater the distortion in your ear, the less you will benefit from amplification, and you may not be able to understand amplified speech by listening alone. That's the bad news. The good news is that even persons with severe hearing loss can learn to benefit substantially from amplified signals and use them along with visual clues to understand speech.

You should look for these things in a hearing-aid evaluation: The recommended aids should make as many speech sounds as possible comfortably loud but not make the loudness of any amplified sound uncomfortable. Hearing aids like this will enable you to use your residual hearing to the best advantage. The following paragraphs give you some suggestions about the processes that help us to search for appropriate amplification.

Who Will Do What to Whom?

Three groups may be involved in helping you select hearing aids: physicians, audiologists, and hearing-aid dispensers. It is possible that at least two of these groups may be represented by the same person. For example, the physician or audiologist who examines you may also sell hearing aids.

The Physician

An ear, nose, and throat specialist or other physician should examine your ears and provide medical clearance for the hearing aid. This examination will establish that your loss is not medically correctable or does not require medical treatment. For example, rarely, hearing loss is caused by a tumor growing on the auditory nerve, a condition which can be life-threatening if not treated.

The Audiologist

You should see an audiologist for hearing evaluation, whose tests can answer three important questions: Do you need hearing aids and if so, how great is the need? Can you benefit from hearing aids, and if so, how much? Finally, what kind of hearing aids do you need?

The Hearing Aid Dispenser

You will need to locate someone to sell you hearing aids at a competitive price, to show you how to use and care for the aids, and to supply follow-up services. These services will include answers to your questions and help with problems which arise as you learn hearing aid use or become acquainted with a new hearing aid. The person who sells the aids to you will also provide warranty service, repair service, and earmold replacement. You should ask about the dispenser's policy regarding trial use. Most dispensers will permit you to return aids after a trial period if you find they do not satisfy your needs. You should also ask about the availability of loaner aids during periods when your own aids must go back to the factory for repairs.

Hearing Aid Selection Strategies

The audiologist who evaluates you will use one of several selection strategies to determine appropriate hearing aids for you. Regardless of the procedure, the following characteristics of the aids selected for you must be determined: **Gain**—how much the aid will increase the level of each sound. Hearing aids are rated according to their maximum gain; that is, gain available when the volume control is turned all the way on. **Maximum power output** (saturation sound pressure level)—the maximum output level that the hearing aid can deliver to your ear regardless of the combination of gain and input sound levels. This limit serves as a safety factor to keep the hearing aid from being uncomfortably loud or harmful to your ear. **Frequency response**—the gain of the aid at different frequencies, from sounds of low pitch to high pitch. Adjusting the frequency response can prevent amplification of frequencies where you have no hearing loss and provide appropriate amplification across frequency as your hearing loss varies. Additional decisions must be made about how the above characteristics will be achieved and about the style of the aids that will be selected. You should know that many aids now on the market have additional controls that offer flexibility in the characteristics mentioned above. This flexibility permits "fine tuning" during your trial use period or even some compensation if your hearing changes during the life of the aid.

During the evaluation, decisions about earmold selection must be made. The basic function of the earmold is to hold the hearing aid in or on your ear without excessive leakage of sound energy. To do this, the earmold must fit well and have sufficient retention capability so that it will not work loose when you talk or chew. An inadequate earmold will let too much amplified sound leak from the ear canal. This sound reenters the hearing-aid microphone, causing a feedback cycle and an unpleasant whistling sound.

Additionally the earmold is sometimes designed to modify acoustic functioning of the aid. The use of vents or openings in the earmold can help you to hear more naturally those sounds for which you have good hearing and reduce unnecessary loudness of some low frequency sounds. Earmolds with acoustic horns enhance high frequency energy. In general, earmolds should be selected to help you achieve your best hearing, not because of concerns about their appearance, and should be of sufficient design to remain in your ear securely.

Essential Components of a State-of-the-Art Hearing Aid Evaluation

Regardless of the evaluation procedures used by your audiologist to select a hearing aid for you, you should look for the following factors in an effective hearing aid evaluation/selection process. The factors are divided into three groups. The first group has to do with the audiologist who evaluates you. The second group concerns the evaluation procedure which will be used. The third group relates to the assistance and service you will get after you have purchased your aids.

Assessor Variables

You should look for the following qualifications in the person who evaluates your hearing and sells hearing aids to you.

Well-trained: Most audiologists hold the Certificate of Clinical Competence awarded by the American Speech-Language-Hearing Association. They ordinarily have at least a Master's degree in Audiology and in most states are licensed to sell hearing aids. Diplomas and documents testifying to these qualifications will ordinarily be posted on office walls. A competent person should not mind your asking about these qualifications.

Well-established: There is an advantage in staying with an established dispenser year after year, who can accumulate records of your hearing impairment, anticipate your needs, and give continuing service. Look for evidence that suggests the person will be there when you need service for your aids or when the time comes to purchase a new aid. You might get clues from the general appearance of the physical plant and furnishings.

Well-equipped: There should be an adequate sound-treated room for your hearing evaluation. If you can hear outside sounds during the test, the room is not adequate. If testing is done with the hearing aid on, the room must be extra quiet, since amplification from the aid will increase the level of outside sounds. Electronic equipment should be available to measure the operating characteristics of your hearing aid. These measures will ensure that the aid meets the manufacturer's specifications, will help the audiologist to make initial settings of the aid, and will detect areas of malfunction. A laboratory where at least minor hearing aid repairs and earmold alterations can be done is helpful.

Competitive prices: Prices for the same hearing aid may vary considerably from dispenser to dispenser. The initial price should not be your only consideration, since the quality of the evaluation, recommendation, and follow-up care are also important. Nevertheless, you may want to check selling price from more than one dispenser. If your dispenser is asking substantially more for your aids, try to establish what additional services are offered for the price.

Warranty/insurance/service: Hearing aids usually carry a one- or two-year warranty. Find out which applies to the aids recommended for you. Many companies sell a third-year warranty which is available for a modest price only at the time you buy the aids. Some companies offer a one-year loss or damage replacement insurance policy at no cost, while others offer this service for a fee. Most companies have a fixed repair charge for routine service to your aid after the warranty period expires. Find out all of this information and get it in writing. As mentioned earlier, you should also get a written statement about the policy for trial use and the availability of loaner aids when yours are in for repair.

Assessment Variables

The following information should be obtained.

Medical clearance: Federal regulations require medical clearance before purchase of an aid, but permit adults eighteen years of age and over to waive this requirement for personal reasons. The dispenser is not permitted to recommend that you waive this requirement, but must tell you that a medical examination is in your best health interests. Even if you have a stable hearing loss from a known and untreatable cause, new problems, detectable by medical examination, may develop. For example, an accumulation of earwax may reduce your hearing further or prevent optimum functioning of your hearing aids. This problem is easily corrected when your doctor removes the wax.

Current complete hearing evaluation: In addition to the information learned about the type of amplification you need, a periodic complete hearing evaluation lets you know if your hearing is changing and alerts your audiologist to developing problems (See Chapter 2). For example, although it happens only rarely, high levels of sound associated with some hearing aids may cause further changes in the hearing of the user. If this problem is detected, the aid can be internally adjusted to a lower power level. For these reasons a complete hearing evalution should precede the fitting of new aids even if your hearing has been tested many times before.

Appropriate aid—type: As you know, hearing aids are available in various types and styles. Very few people wear body-type hearing aids nowadays. Until recently, behind-the-ear aids were most popular and they deliver efficient and flexible service, especially to people with severe losses. Currently, in the United States, the majority of hearing aid sales are of in-the-ear or in-the-canal aids. While there are some disadvantages to these aids, they operate well for many hearing losses. The most important point is this: your aids should be recommended to provide you with best hearing function, rather than entirely for cosmetic reasons. That is, while you want hearing aids that look as nice as possible, you should not sacrifice function for appearance. Before permanently accepting in-the-ear or in-the-canal aids, you should be sure you can get as much loudness as you need without feedback and that the aids will remain securely in your ears. The ears of some individuals are too small to accommodate in-the-ear or in-the-canal aids. Additionally, you may need certain features that are not currently available on in-the-ear or in-the-canal aids. For example, it is not always possible to build strong telephone coils into them. Also, jacks for the insertion of external microphones are not always available in these aids, so they may not give you best possible hearing in noisy places or large rooms. See chapters 5 and 6 on assistive listening devices for detailed discussion of these advantages. If you need these features, behind-the-ear aids are ordinarily the instruments of choice.

Appropriate aid—operating characteristics: You deserve careful evaluation of the function of your new aids on your ear. The aids should be selected and adjusted to permit comfortable hearing of as many speech sounds as possible. This process requires an evaluation which may continue over several sessions, as the experiences you report indicate the need for additional adjustment.

Follow-up Variables

Making the bad good, or what if the dispenser goofs? During the trial-use period, problems may arise which the good dispenser will try to correct. As just mentioned, the dispenser should be willing and able to adjust your aids, in response to problems which you report, for more effective, comfortable amplification. Occasionally, however, inappropriate aids may be recommended, especially in difficult-to-fit cases. To insist that this should never happen would probably reduce the tendency to try unconventional fittings which may provide the best amplification or even to recommend an aid at all in borderline candidates for amplification. In cases where the selection turns out not to work well after thorough trial, the good supplier will be willing to try again. And if all efforts fail, the aid should be returnable under terms that you should ascertain before purchase. These terms may justifiably include nonrefundable fees for the dispenser's services, the earmold, and perhaps a rental fee for the time you had the aids.

The fit of a new earmold is sometimes inadequate. It may be too loose and cause excessive feedback or be uncomfortable because it doesn't fit well. Some modification of earmolds to improve fit can be done by your dispenser, although these changes are limited with in-the-ear and in-the-canal aids, which ordinarily fit into the earmold. The good dispenser will be willing to stay with the problem until it is corrected and order a new earmold at no charge if it is necessary. If an earmold hurts, don't wait. See your dispenser immediately.

Instruction and support: If you are a veteran hearing aid user, the instruction you need may be limited to orienting you to the operation of a different set of controls on your new hearing aids. However, new users (and some previous hearing aid wearers) have much to learn about the care, operation, and optimum use of amplification. The good dispenser will teach these skills and support you during the sometimes difficult process of adjusting to amplification. Find out the dispenser's policy about return visits before your purchase.

Availability: You should buy your aids from a dispenser who can help you promptly when you have trouble. Find out about the dispenser's policy: working hours, whether an appointment is required, how long you may have to wait if you drop in, and turnaround time for repairs.

Summary

A hearing aid is a tiny efficient amplifier. It increases the level of sounds so that you can hear them. How well you can understand the amplified sounds depends on the status of your ear, selection of appropriate hearing aids, and whether or not you have learned to use the aids optimally.

You can improve your odds for success by taking good medical and audiologic care of your ears. Medical clearance should precede hearing aid use, and regular ear examinations are also important. Thorough and regular hearing evaluations are essential to your hearing, to the selection and maintenance of appropriate hearing aids, and to your best chance for success in college. Your audiologist may recommend these checkups about once a year, or sooner if problems are noted. Your audiologist will conduct a hearing aid evaluation to select the operating characteristics of your new hearing aids. Decisions will be made to select appropriate gain, maximum output, style, and other characteristics for best performance.

You should select a hearing aid dispenser who is adequately trained and equipped, who will provide appropriate amplification, show you how to use it well, and be available to give you good follow-up service when you have questions or your hearing aids need service. On the next page there appears a check list you should take along when you venture forth to seek your next hearing aids.

Hearing Aid Selection Check List

( ) Qualified, well-trained dispenser. Certified by the American Speech-Language-Hearing Association and/or licensed by your state.

(   ) Well-established dispenser. Someone who has been in business for a time and seems likely to be there when you need service or new hearing aids.

(   ) Well-equipped. Your dispenser should have adequate equipment for valid hearing and hearing-aid evaluation, as well as for hearing aid analysis and repair.

(   ) Competitive prices. Ascertain that, consistent with services offered, your dispenser charges the rates prevailing in your community.

(   ) Warranty/insurance/service. Learn the details about these important areas.

(   ) Medical clearance form signed by an otolaryngologist or other physician to certify that hearing aid use is not contraindicated for medical reasons.

(   ) Audiological evaluation including:
   A. Pure tone air and bone conduction thresholds which indicate how much and what kind of hearing loss you have. This information reveals whether you have any potentially correctable (conductive) hearing loss, how much you need amplification in terms of the magnitude of your loss, and provides important information to determine the gain and frequency response of your aids.
   B. Word recognition ability. These tests tell about your ability to differentiate speech sounds and provide an idea of how much benefit you may expect from amplification. Testing in background noise as well as in quiet may give additional information about your hearing aid candidacy and the type of amplification required.
   C. Tests which establish most comfortable and uncomfortably loud listening levels. This information helps to select hearing aid characteristics that provide effective, comfortable listening.

(   ) Style of aids. In selecting behind-the-ear vs. in-the-ear aids you should consider:
   A. The options you need, such as strong telecoils or jacks for plugging in external microphones. These options may not be available in in-the-ear aids.
   B. Gain, particularly in the high frequency areas. There may be more feedback problems with in-the-ear aids, and the problems are routinely solved by reducing high frequency gain, which may reduce your aids' effectiveness.

(   ) Appropriate earmold. Your molds should be appropriately styled to prevent feedback. They should be designed for sound quality and comfort. Cosmetics, an important concern, should not preempt function.

( ) Follow-up services. Make sure your dispenser will be available when you need assistance, warranty service, or hearing aid repairs. Find out if a trial period of use is available, during which your aids can be adjusted as needed or even returned if they are unsatisfactory.

Suggestions for Further Reading

Gauger, J., Clymer, E., Young, M., and Woolever L., *Orientation to Hearing Aids.* Rochester: National Technical Institute for the Deaf (undated). Available from: The Alexander Graham Bell Association for the Deaf, 3417 Volta Place, N.W., Washington, DC 20007. In simple language and step-by-step fashion, this set of booklets explains what hearing aids are and what they do, earmolds and hearing-aid batteries, maintenance and care of hearing aids, troubleshooting hearing aid problems, and gives consumer information about hearing aids.

Hodgson, W. (ed.), *Hearing Aid Assessment and Use in Audiologic Habilitation* (3rd. ed.). Baltimore: Williams and Wilkins (1986). Intended as a college text, this book may be helpful to those who want to read in more depth or get more technical information about hearing aid assessment and use.

Rezen, S., and Hausman, C., *Coping with Hearing Loss.* New York: Dembner Books (1985). Written for hearing impaired adults and their families, this book contains general information about hearing and hearing loss as well as ways to cope with hearing loss, including the selection and use of hearing aids.

SHHH, Self Help for Hard of Hearing People, Inc., 7800 Wisconsin Ave., Bethesda, MD 20814. In addition to information about new aspects of hearing aids and hearing aid use, this monthly magazine contains informative and supportive articles about all aspects of hearing loss.

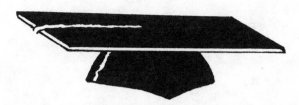

PART II-REHABILITATION

Now that the students, their hearing losses, and appropriate hearing aids have been identified, how can we best address the demands imposed by a college environment? This section of the book has been an attempt to draw together all of those seemingly elusive bits of critical survival information from several different disciplines.

Chapter 4 emphasizes the type of hearing aid fitting most suited for the unique demands of college communication. However, as discussed in Chapter 5, the student with hearing loss must go beyond hearing aids and utilize a variety of assistive communication devices in order to be competitive with hearing peers. Chapter 6 details the fickle nature of classroom listening as well as the means available for environmental control. Vocational Rehabilitation Services may provide the ticket to college for many students who are hearing impaired; and Chapter 7 is an excellent presentation of how to understand and effectively use this wonderful service. Chapter 8 is a compendium of practical information ranging from how to select a college to a listing of services/accommodations available through the Office of Student Services for the Handicapped. Chapter 9 tells how a student can get help in order to learn how to learn. Chapter 10 dispels the myth that a college-aged student with hearing loss has outgrown his/her need for the speech-language pathologist; and Chapter 11 describes oral interpreting, the newest support service.

Thus, the "Rehabilitation" section of this book provides a wealth of need-to-know information compiled from a variety of resources. Knowledge of available sources of help allows the student with hearing loss to be in charge of his/her college experience rather than being unintentionally victimized.

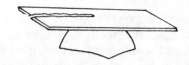

Chapter 4
Isn't One Hearing Aid as Good as Another?

Ron Leavitt, M.S.

Today's college students who are hearing impaired have an opportunity to do something that was not possible twenty years ago. Today, these students have the opportunity to communicate adequately in educational and social situations *if* they are willing to pay the price. Impossible, you say? Read on!

When I first started working at Western Oregon State College, I met thirteen students with hearing impairments and invited them to my office. I asked if they would be willing to experiment with some new assistive listening devices. Interestingly, many of these students said they were doing fine and did not need any new technology. I thought this was strange, since most of them had obsolete hearing aids that were always whistling, and all were wearing white earmolds that I thought were unattractive. One freshman student who used black tape on her earmold to keep the tubing from falling off said she would like some new tubing. I fixed her tubing and told her that I could get her an earmold that was clear rather than white. She agreed to this, and before too long she replaced her old hearing aids. Similarly, all thirteen students eventually changed to the clear earmold material, started using more up-to-date hearing aids, and obtained a variety of other technology that helps them succeed in college. This other technology is described in more detail in Chapter 5.

Now, when I say to these thirteen students that they can communicate in any educational or personal setting, they agree. In fact, several of these students travel throughout Washington and Oregon telling other people with hearing impairments about the possibilities of communicating adequately in every listening situation by making better use of technology.

The point of this story is that most college students with hearing impairments that I have met in the past thirteen years thought they were "doing fine" and that they did not need the information presented in this book. Yet I have never met a student who is aware of the full range of technology available, or who is familiar with the federal regulations requiring use and funding of such equipment. Not having the information presented in this book has cost many students thousands of dollars in misdirected educational programs. So keep reading. What you learn will change your life, as it has for the students who wrote Chapter 15.

The first thing you need to know is that to make successful use of any technology, there is a "price" to pay. In Chapters 12 and 15, we will discuss what that means. For now, we will discuss the technical information about hearing aid success. In Chapter 5 we will discuss other essential technology.

Hearing Aid Considerations

You should know that the hearing aid is one of the most misunderstood pieces of equipment in the world. Most college students do *not* understand what makes their hearing aid whistle, or how to use the telephone switch on their hearing aid. This is unfortunate, since a whistling hearing aid does not work well. Furthermore, proper use of the hearing aid's telephone switch makes it possible for some students with hearing impairment to hear better than their normal-hearing friends in some situations (Bankoski & Ross, 1984). We have also discovered several other things that students need to know about hearing aids so that they can communicate adequately in educational and personal situations. These items are listed below:

Item 1. The Hearing Aid Is Like a Very Small Public Address System.

As noted in Chapter 3, the hearing aid has a microphone that changes sound into electrical energy, an amplifier that increases the electrical energy from the microphone, a battery that provides power for the amplifier, an earphone that changes the amplified energy back into sound, a volume wheel that controls how much amplification the hearing aid provides, an on-off and telephone switch, and other internal controls which we will describe later. There is also a piece of plastic, silicone or polyvinyl chloride, which is form-fit to each student's ear. This form-fit plastic and the tubing that runs through it are called an earmold. Although much has been written about hearing aids, it is perhaps the earmold which recently has been researched the most. For a more detailed technical discussion of the electrical components of the hearing aid, the interested reader is referred to Olsen's excellent article (Olsen, 1986). A technical discussion of the earmold is also available elsewhere (Leavitt, 1986). For now, it's sufficient to know that a properly fitted earmold does not allow the hearing aid to whistle on its normal volume setting. Further, the earmold should not hurt the ear. If ear pain does occur from the earmold, see your audiologist for possible earmold adjustment or your doctor if a medical problem is causing the ear pain.

All five types of hearing aids shown in Chapter 3 have most of these same components. The differences among them are quite small when you consider sound quality. However, some of the smaller in-the-ear aids and all of the in-the-canal aids are too small for a telephone switch, or highly flexible internal controls. If, after reading this chapter, you decide you want a telephone switch and all of the internal controls described later, in-the-canal aids may not be for you.

Item 2. No College Student Who Is Hard-of-Hearing Should Obtain a Hearing Aid Without a Complete Medical, Hearing, and Hearing Aid Evaluation.

This has been discussed in Chapters 2 and 3 and will not be discussed further. Suffice it to say that if you do not get a comprehensive hearing and hearing aid test from an audiologist with the most up-to-date equipment, you may not get the latest technology on your hearing aid. As a result, you will not achieve your best possible hearing.

Item 3. Two Hearing Aids Are Better than One.

Although some college students have one ear that is too impaired to use a hearing aid, most can benefit from two hearing aids. Two hearing aids make it easier to understand speech in noisy places and to identify the location of incoming sound (see Ross, 1977 for further discussion). Additionally, a person with two hearing aids can hear when someone speaks softly from either side. So, unless you have one ear that is too impaired for a hearing aid, you should wear two.

Item 4. Hearing Aids with Directional Microphones Improve Speech Understanding in Noise.

Today's hearing aids can reduce background noise by use of a device called a directional microphone. Since most college students listen in noisy places much of the time (Gengel, 1981), it is a good idea to have a hearing aid that can reduce background noise. Although these directional microphones do *not* eliminate background noise, they give the hearing aid wearer a better chance of understanding speech in noisy places.

One student with a severe hearing loss, who is now an audiologist, told me that directional microphones on her hearing aids help her in noisy places as much as using her second hearing aid. This has now been supported by research (Hawkins & Yacullo, 1984). For this reason, most students who are hard-of-hearing at Western Oregon State College (WOSC) use directional microphones on their hearing aids, except when such a microphone is not available on the model of hearing aid they want.

Item 5. Every Hearing Aid Should Have Internal Controls That Can Change the Amplifying Characteristics of the Hearing Aid.

State-of-the-art hearing aids can be fine-tuned to each person's hearing loss. At WOSC, most students have needed some hearing aid adjustment after their initial fitting. For this reason, it is important that hearing aids have controls which allow the audiologist to make the following adjustments:

1. amplification of soft and moderately loud sounds (called an acoustic gain control);
2. amplification limiting for very loud sounds (called saturation sound pressure level or SSPL control);
3. amplification of low-pitched sounds (called a low-frequency control or a low-frequency trimmer);
4. amplification of high-pitched sounds (called a high-frequency control or a high-frequency trimmer); and
5. automatic volume controls, which automatically reduce the hearing aid's volume when loud sounds occur.

As mentioned earlier, most in-the-ear and in-the-canal hearing aids do not offer all of these internal controls at present. If you want all these options, a behind-the-ear hearing aid is preferred.

Item 6. Hearing Aids Should Provide Adequate Amplification of Low- and High-Pitched Sounds.

Research has shown that people with mild and moderate hearing losses understand speech more clearly when their hearing aids amplify a wide range of high- and low-pitched sounds. This is because the high-pitched sounds in our language, like *s, z, sh, ch, th, f, p,* and *k,* are very important to speech understanding. If the hearing aid cannot amplify these sounds to a level that the student can hear, it is unlikely these words will be understood. Thus, students with mild and moderate hearing losses and even those with severe hearing losses in the 85 dB range or better at 2000, 4000, and 6000 Hz should ask for hearing aids that provide this high-fidelity amplification. This way, all high-pitched sounds will be amplified to a level that is audible. It is important to realize, however, that having these sounds amplified does not guarantee complete speech understanding. For complete speech understanding to occur, the brain must interpret sound into meaningful sentences. If the ear's function is too severely impaired, speech understanding will not occur and sound enhancement technology described in Chapter 5, speech reading (lipreading), educated guessing, and perhaps sign language will be required.

Item 7. Hearing Aids Must Be Connected to Appropriate Earmold Tubing.

About eighteen years ago, a hearing aid engineer suggested that the tubes that connect body aids, eyeglass aids, and behind-the-ear hearing aids to the ear should be carefully chosen so that they would not interfere with the amplification provided by the hearing aid (Lybarger, 1972). Unfortunately, many hearing aids have been fitted without appropriate tubing (Flexer, Wray & Black, 1986). As a result, some of the high-pitched amplification provided by today's hearing aids has been lost. In other instances, inappropriate use of tubing can create a whistling sound in the hearing aid which is known as acoustic feedback. Although appropriate tubing selection is too complicated to discuss here, a detailed discussion is available elsewhere (Leavitt, 1985).

For the purpose of this chapter, one simple rule applies: maximum high-pitched amplification *cannot* be provided from a behind-the-ear hearing aid unless the tubing in the earmold gets bigger as it enters the ear canal. If the earmold tubing is the same size all the way from the hearing aid to the tip of the earmold, you are not getting the most high-pitched amplification possible. If you feel you could benefit from this high-pitched amplification, ask your audiologist about some of this special earmold tubing.

Item 8. Hearing Aids Should Be Equipped with High-Fidelity Telephone Switches.

Body aids, eyeglass aids, behind-the-ear aids, and many in-the-ear aids can be equipped with a special switch called a telephone or "T" switch. While the hearing aid is set to its telephone position, a coil of wire inside the hearing aid receives the magnetic signals produced by the telephone earpiece. When the telephone switch is turned on, the hearing aid will only respond to these magnetic signals. Thus, by turning on the telephone switch, a student with hearing aids can reduce background noise, which is regular acoustic sound, and listen only to the magnetic sound produced by the telephone.

Oftentimes, when I have mentioned telephone switches, students report that they hear adequately on the telephone with their built-in telephone amplifiers, and do not need a telephone switch on their hearing aids. However, as stated earlier, the hearing aid's telephone switch also provides a way of reducing background noise. This "noise reducing" function is accomplished by an electromagnetic induction loop system. Without a telephone switch on the hearing aid the loop cannot be used to reduce noise. Research has shown that reducing background noise is the single most important consideration when providing hearing assistance to people with hearing difficulty (Leavitt & Hodgson, 1982). For this reason, a telephone switch is strongly recommended. Additionally, it is important to have the audiologist check the hearing aid's telephone switch to see that it is working properly. Such testing is not routinely performed, but is essential for the effective use of the loop system.

Item 9. Earmolds Must Fit Properly.

Whether the student uses a body aid, eyeglass aid, behind-the-ear aid, in-the-ear aid, or in-the-canal aid, there must be some way of fitting the hearing aid on the ear. This form-fitting device is called an earmold. It is essential that this device fit properly. If proper fit is not achieved, the ear becomes sore and, in some instances, painful lesions develop. If too much sound leaks out around the earmold and gets back into the microphone of the hearing aid, the bothersome whistling sound called acoustic feedback occurs. When feedback occurs, attention is drawn to the hearing aid. Further, the whistling hearing aid cannot function properly. Thus if there is ear pain, or if the hearing aid is whistling, the earmold and aid should be checked by an audiologist. Invariably, both ear pain and feedback can be reduced and often eliminated.

Item 10. Hearing Aids Should Provide High-Fidelity Amplification.

In addition to amplifying a wide range of pitches, the hearing aid should provide a fairly accurate reproduction of speech. In other words, if a sound in the environment has equal energy at all pitches between 500 and 4000 Hz, then after this sound has been amplified by the hearing aid, there should be no large differences in how the pitches between 500 and 4000 Hz are amplified (Killion & Tillman, 1982; Libby, 1981). The best way for an audiologist to test for this "smooth amplification" is by using a computerized measurement system. Although some research has questioned whether hearing aid users prefer this type of amplification (Cox & Alexander, 1983), there is no doubt that this equal amplification principle helps control feedback. Further, some research suggests equal amplification improves speech understanding (Jerger & Thelin, 1968; Libby, 1981; Soeholt, 1983). If a hearing aid does not provide this type of equal amplification when connected to the ear, there are a variety of things the audiologist can do. If your hearing aid is not providing relatively accurate sound reproduction, ask if such a hearing aid fitting can be made.

Item 11. Earmold Venting Should Be Used when Appropriate.

Many students have relatively normal hearing for low-pitched sounds, with most of their hearing impairment in the high-pitched range. For these students, low-pitch sounds should not be amplified by the hearing aid. To prevent this amplification of low pitches, the internal controls of the hearing aid can be adjusted. However, research has shown that adjusting the hearing aid's internal controls to limit amplification of low pitches often produces a less pleasing sound quality (Cox & Alexander, 1983). The same reduction of low-pitched energy can be achieved by drilling a hole, known as a vent, into the earmold. Research has shown that better sound quality is often achieved by venting than by modifying the hearing aid's internal controls. Additionally, the vent helps to keep the ear cooler, although feedback can be a problem if the vent is too large. At Western Oregon State College when a student can benefit from an earmold vent, a positive venting valve (PVV) is ordered. This PVV allows the audiologist to quickly adjust the size of the vent to control feedback while allowing for maximum reduction of low-pitched amplification.

Numerous college students with high-pitched hearing losses are now using vents. More detailed information on earmold venting is available elsewhere (Leavitt, 1986).

Item 12. Hearing Aids That Change Their Amplifying Characteristics when Background Noise Is Present Should Be Considered.

Within the last few years, it has become possible for hearing aids to change their amplification when background noise is present. The idea behind such a "changeable" hearing aid is that background noise is mostly low-pitched. Thus, a hearing aid that reduces low-pitched amplification in noise and boosts high-pitched speech energy should have the effect of reducing noise. Unfortunately, many speech sounds are low-pitched, so when low-pitched amplification is reduced in a noisy place, some of the speech that you want to hear will also be lost (Van Tassel, Larsen, & Fabry, 1987). As a result, students who use these changeable hearing aids continue to experience difficulty hearing in a noisy classroom because the typical classroom dramatically changes the teacher's voice as it travels from the teacher to the student's ear (Leavitt & Flexer, 1990). For students with hearing loss, this sound alteration creates communication problems. So, even when a "changeable" hearing aid is used, the student will still need a hardwire, frequency-modulation (FM), infrared, or loop system such as described in Chapter 5 to achieve the best possible hearing in the classroom. Students and educators must not rely solely on high-fidelity, state-of-the-art hearing aids to provide optimum sound reception (Leavitt & Flexer, 1990).

Item 13. Earmolds Should Be Cosmetically Acceptable.

The first twelve items suggest ways to improve communication ability. This suggestion is made to enhance a student's personal appearance. While students with hearing aids should not try to hide their hearing loss (see Chapter 12 for further discussion), there should not be an unnecessary cosmetic penalty for having a hearing loss. This means that students should choose earmolds that are cosmetically acceptable to them. Many people wear white earmolds because they are not aware that clear earmolds exist. Others have been told that there was less chance of allergic reaction with white earmold material. Yet allergic reaction to the soft clear earmold material called polyvinyl chloride is rare.

This lack of allergic reaction to clear material is not surprising since the tubing in every earmold is polyvinyl chloride and allergic reaction to the tubing rarely occurs. So, when it's time for a new earmold, ask for an earmold color that is cosmetically appealing. At WOSC, this usually means the hard, clear lucite earmold material is used by students with mild to moderate hearing losses, except those who are active in sports. Soft, clear polyvinyl chloride earmolds are used by all others to assure maximum feedback protection and to protect the ear during activities where the ear may be accidentally bumped.

Item 14. Earmold Tubing Should Be Designed to Prevent Moisture Condensation Inside the Tubing.

Whether a student lives in a humid area or in a hot desert, condensation of moisture inside the tubing of the earmold is a problem. At worst, this moisture can damage the hearing aid, or plug the filters placed in the hearing aid's earhook causing the hearing aid to stop working. For this reason, students who use eyeglass or behind-the-ear hearing aids should ask for "Dri-tubes" in their earmold. Dri tubes prevent moisture condensation in the earmold tubing and help to protect the hearing aid. They are only a few dollars more than the regular tubing and worth the investment.

By using these fourteen suggestions, all students with hearing impairment at WOSC have improved their ability to hear and understand speech in the classroom. Additionally, their hearing aids do not whistle every time they smile or chew; and they do not have highly visible earmolds. In my experience, these last two improvements have been, in some instances, as important as improved hearing in the classroom.

Finally, it must be remembered that using all fourteen of these suggestions for improved hearing aid fittings will not provide optimum hearing in the classroom or any other difficult listening situation. A hardwire, FM, infrared, or loop system must also be used. These systems are discussed in the next two chapters and are necessary for optimum classroom hearing. So, read on and discover some additional essential technology.

References

Bankoski, S.M., & Ross, M. (1984). FM systems' effect on speech discrimination in an auditorium. *Hearing Instruments, 35,* 8.

Cox, R., & Alexander, C. (1983). Acoustic versus electronic modifications of hearing aid low-frequency output. *Ear and Hearing, 4,* 190–196.

Flexer, C., Wray, D.F., & Black, T.S. (1986). Support group for moderately hearing impaired college students: An expanding awareness. *The Volta Review, 88,* 223–229.

Gengel, R. (1981). Acceptable signal-to-noise ratios for aided speech discrimination by the hearing impaired. *Journal of Auditory Research, 11,* 219–222.

Hawkins, D.B., & Yacullo, W.S. (1984). Signal-to-noise ratio advantages of binaural hearing aids and directional microphones under different levels of reverberation. *Journal of Speech and Hearing Disorders, August,* 278–286.

Jerger, J. & Thelin, J. (1968). Effects of electroacoustic characteristics of hearing aids on speech understanding. *Bulletin of Prosthetics Research, 11,* 159–197.

Killion, M. & Tillman, T. (1982). Evaluation of high-fidelity hearing aids. *Journal of Speech and Hearing Research, 25,* 15–25.

Leavitt, R.J. (1985). Counseling to encourage the use of SNR enhancing systems. *Hearing Instruments, 36,* 8–9.

Leavitt, R.J. (1986). Earmolds: acoustic and structural considerations. In W.R. Hodgson (Ed.) *Hearing Aid Assessment and Use in Audiologic Habilitation: Third Edition,* Chapter 4. Baltimore: Williams & Wilkins.

Leavitt, R.J. (1987). Promoting the use of rehabilitation technology. *ASHA, 29,* 28–31.

Leavitt, R.J., & Flexer, C.A. (1990). Speech degradation in a typical listening environment as measured by the Rapid Speech Transmission Index (RASTI). Proceedings of the Annual American Academy of Audiology Convention, New Orleans, Louisiana.

Leavitt, R.J., & Hodgson, W.R. (1982). Use of radio-frequency amplifying systems vs. binaural hearing aids. Proceedings of the Annual American Speech-Language and Hearing Association Convention, Toronto, Canada.

Libby, E. (1981). Achieving a transparent, smooth, wide-band hearing aid response. *Hearing Instruments, 32,* 9.

Lybarger, S.F. (1972). Earmolds. In J. Katz (Ed.). *Handbook of Clinical Audiology,* Chapter 32, Baltimore: Williams and Wilkins.

Olsen, W.O. (1986). Physical characteristics of hearing aids. In W.R. Hodgson (Ed.). *Hearing Aid Assessment and Use in Audiologic Habilitation: Third Edition,* Chapter 4. Baltimore: Williams and Wilkins.

Ross, M. (1977). Binaural vs. monaural hearing amplification for hearing impaired individuals. In Bess, F. (Ed.). *Childhood Deafness: Detection, Assessment and Management,* Chapter 19. Orlando, FL: Grune and Stratton.

Soeholt, F. (1983). Earmolds with horn bores. *Hearing Instruments, 34,* 17.

Van Tassel, D.J., Larsen, S.Y. & Fabry, D.A. (1987). Speech recognition in noise with an adaptive filter hearing aid. Proceedings of the annual Speech-Language and Hearing Association Convention, New Orleans, Louisiana.

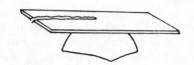

Chapter 5
Beyond Hearing Aids: The Mystical World of Assistive Communication Devices

Carol Flexer, Ph.D.,
Frederick S. Berg, Ph.D.

What would it be like to sit in school classrooms for twelve years and hear little of the lectures and discussions? To attend business meetings yet not be sure of the final decision? To be deprived of the enjoyment of leisure conversation in a restaurant? To not "catch" TV or movie or play dialogue? To not hear the keynote address in professional meetings? To feel anxious when speaking over the phone and in fact to avoid such communication? To not quite understand the minister's sermon? And to feel isolated in social gatherings? Twenty million Americans with hearing loss know exactly what it is like.

The number of personal and professional sacrifices that a person with hearing loss must make is appalling (Diedrichsen, 1987; Leavitt, 1985, 1987; Vaughn, 1986). No other disability would tolerate such lack of accessibility to societal interactions. Unfortunately, most persons who are hearing impaired, including college students, are not aware of alternatives which would open the doors of communication. The hearing aid has been viewed as the only technology available, and when the aid is ineffective in certain environments (as it surely will be), the person who is hearing impaired is at a complete loss. Therefore, the purpose of this chapter is to discuss the range of communication devices which could provide accessibility to the social and business communication scenarios mentioned above. People with hearing loss need not live life on the fringe!

Why Isn't a Hearing Aid Enough?

Hearing aids, as discussed in detail in Chapters 3 and 4 of this book, have never been able to provide "easy listening" in all environments. Reasons for this lack of perfection include the properties of the hearing aid, the type of listening environment, and the damaged ear of the listener. **These difficulties generally pertain to the concept of signal-to-noise ratio (S/N); the relationship between the signal that the listener wishes to hear and all other irrelevant sounds.**

A person who has a hearing loss, even when wearing a hearing aid, requires a more favorable S/N in order to understand speech than does a person with normal hearing. That is, most people with normal hearing can easily understand the speaker when the signal of choice is twice as loud as background sounds. Unfortunately, persons with hearing losses require the signal of choice to be ten times louder than background sounds before it can be clearly understood (Berg, 1986). Such a favorable S/N is impossible to obtain in a large area, in noisy environments, or when the desired signal is some distance from the listener. In short, an effective S/N cannot be obtained in any classroom (see Chapter 6 for elaboration), church, auditorium, theater, or outdoors.

Thus, hearing aids, appropriately fitted, can be very effective for communicating in relatively quiet environments where the speaker is close to the listener. In addition, hearing aids can enhance "audibility" from a distance. However, for adequate "intelligibility," a favorable S/N is imperative, with such a S/N typically requiring that the hearing aid's function be augmented or enhanced by assistive communication devices.

What Are Assistive Communication Devices?

Leavitt (1987) felt that the term "Rehabilitation Technology for People with Hearing Loss" was appropriately descriptive and, accordingly divided available communication devices into four categories: sound enhancement technology, television enhancement technology, telecommunication technology, and signal alerting technology. **Don't let the word "technology" scare you off, because all of this equipment logically functions to make the signal of choice more "intelligible" to the listener who is hearing impaired.** The categories are descriptive because they divide equipment by intended use according to the needs of the individual. That is, the person with hearing loss can select, from many options, those pieces of equipment that can most directly address his/ her communication needs.

Following will be a brief discussion of available equipment as categorized above. In addition, addresses and phone numbers of national manufacturers will be presented at the end of this chapter. College students are advised to contact their audiologist or their university's speech and hearing clinic for detailed information and hands-on practice with equipment. Also, the New York League for the Hard-of-Hearing (address and phone number at the end of this chapter) has produced an informative videotape about assistive devices as well as serving as a national resource for information about available technology.

Sound Enhancement Technology

Also called Assistive Listening Devices (ALD), sound enhancement technology enables the person with hearing loss to hear speech clearly in large or noisy rooms by essentially bypassing the unfavorable environment and transmitting the signal directly to the listener (Ross, 1986). All ALD's work on the principle of a **remote microphone** which can be placed close to the sound source, thereby avoiding the weakening of the speech signal as it travels some distance from the speaker to the listener. If the listener could personally be very close to the speaker, then this remote microphone might not be necessary. However, in many group situations (e.g., classrooms, lecture halls, theaters, churches, noisy restaurants) the listener simply cannot get close enough to the speaker to have the speech be intelligible (to hear each speech sound as clearly distinct from another). So, a microphone, attached to some type of transmitter, functions to provide a good S/N. **Thus, the positioning of this remote microphone close to the sound source (usually within six inches) is the secret of the success of ALD's.**

1. Personal and Group FM (Frequency Modulation) Systems

FM is a term applied to the radio transmission of signals whereby speech, after being changed into an electrical signal, is superimposed on a radio signal which is then transmitted (Berg, 1987). In 1982, the Federal Communications Commission (FCC) authorized the use of the 72-76 MHZ band for use by persons with hearing loss not only in classrooms, but also in other difficult listening conditions.

Using an FM system is like having your own tiny, private radio station that sends or transmits (speaker), and receives (listener) on a

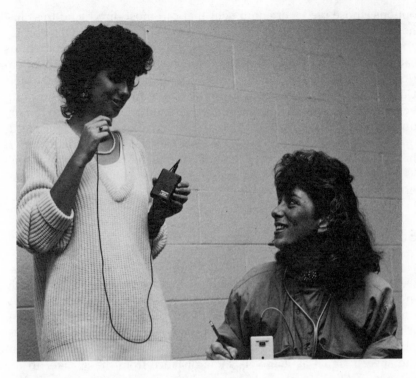

**Figure 5-1: An FM System Is Like Having Your Own Tiny, Private Radio
Station That Transmits and Receives on a Single Frequency.**

single frequency. The speaker and listener are not connected by wires,
allowing free mobility up to the range of the equipment, usually about
200 feet. The transmission is generally free from interference, providing
that no other units are using the same frequency in the same environment. The cost of FM equipment varies from approximately $500 to $1200
for a single transmitter and receiver. (Figure 5-1)

The FM receiver can send the signal to the listener's ear through
one of several options: use of an earpiece which is connected from the
receiver to the listener's ear by a wire (that is, the listener removes his/
her hearing aid and inserts the earpiece or puts on headphones); a wire
or loop worn around the listener's neck which, when connected to the
receiver, generates a magnetic field that is picked up by the "T" attach-
ment on the listener's hearing aid (provided that the listener's aid is
equipped with an appropriate "T" or telephone coil); or a direct input
cord which, through electrical input, connects the FM receiver to the
hearing aid (see Chapter 6 for pictures and more detail).

The listener can easily carry both transmitter and receiver of a personal FM unit with him/her and give the transmitter to the desired speaker in any situation. For example, a college student who is hard-of-hearing might have his/her own FM unit of which the transmitter is handed to the professor prior to the start of class to enable the student, who is wearing the receiver, to more clearly hear the lecture.

A skeptical graduate student, who had been moderately hearing impaired since birth, tried an FM unit to prove that he didn't need it in class. He raced back from the lecture in a state of astonishment. "I can't believe it!" he said. "I didn't know that professors didn't mumble. I didn't know that it was possible to take notes and listen at the same time. I didn't know that I could leave class without being totally exhausted and dripping wet from concentrating so hard. I didn't know that I didn't have to guess at what the professor really 'meant.' I didn't know that I could still follow the lecture when the professor turned his back to write on the board. I didn't know that I could still hear over the hum of the slide projector. This unit is really a 'clarifier' because it makes speech so clear and easy to hear." Now, in our college support group, FM units have become known as "clarifiers."

Group FM systems may be installed in a large meeting place with multiple receivers available to be "checked-out" by listeners, each set to the same frequency to pick up the signal from a single transmitter. For example, a church might have an FM system put in, with the pastor wearing a single FM transmitter, and perhaps twenty receivers being available to parishioners who are hearing impaired.

2. Induction Loop System

The loop system has a long wire which is either temporarily placed or permanently installed around a room or specific seating area. This wire generates a magnetic field when connected to a special amplifier that receives the signal from a microphone which is placed near the speaker or sound source (Leavitt & Hodgson, 1984). The listener with hearing loss must have a good quality "T" (telephone) switch on his/her hearing aid in order to take advantage of a loop system. In addition, the listener must sit within the circle of the wire placed around the room (Smith, 1985).

The loop system can be installed in the individual's home (in a specific room), in classrooms, or in larger places like churches or theaters. While not as practical or portable as FM systems, they can accommodate a larger number of persons with hearing loss within a single room (provided that they all have quality "T" attachments on their hearing aids) for less money, approximately $130 for a small unit.

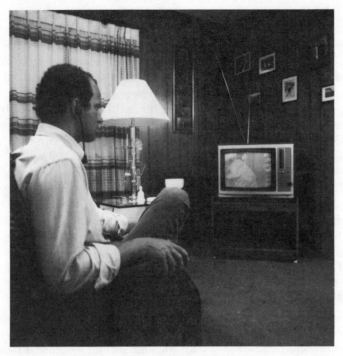

Figure 5-2: An Infrared System Transmits Sound on Light Waves.

3. Infrared Systems

Infrared systems must be used indoors within a single room, because they use the transmission medium of invisible light, the wavelength of which is outside the range of human visibility. The unit consists of a remote microphone placed near the desired speaker (or sound source) which sends the signal to a transmitter. The transmitter, often physically placed high in the room, emits a signal consisting of lightwaves that spread throughout the room (Wayner, 1986). The message from the sound source carried on these lightwaves is picked up by a special stethoscope-like receiver worn by the listener. Infrared systems offer good quality sound for concerts, lectures, theatre, radio, and TV. They are wireless, and cost varies from about $150 for a personal transmitter and receiver, to about $2500 for a unit powerful enough to accommodate a large auditorium. (Figure 5-2)

4. Hardwire Systems

Hardwire systems are so named because the speaker and listener are physically connected to one another by actual wires. The remote

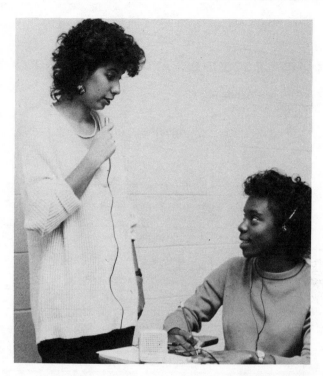

Figure 5-3: When Using a Hardwire System, the Sound Is Transmitted Through Connecting Wires Rather than Via Radio Waves or Light Waves.

microphone is placed next to the speaker (within the limitations of the length of the connecting wire) with a connecting wire to an amplifier. The sound amplifier is also connected by wire to headphones or earpiece worn by the listener. While obviously restricting mobility, hardwire units can be very useful for one-to-one communication situations, such as individual speech/language therapy (Sudler & Flexer, 1986), talking in a car, restaurants, patient interviews and counseling (Wayner, 1986), and television viewing (Figure 5-3). Hardwire units can be relatively inexpensive (starting about $50) because they can be assembled from easily obtained parts (Vaughn, Lightfoot, & Gibbs, 1983).

To assist the reader in evaluating the qualities and determining the relevance of each type of ALD for his/her individual needs, Figure 5-4 is included.

Television-Enhancement Technology

All of the sound enhancement technology mentioned previously can be used with television and video systems. The remote microphone

SUMMARY OF SOUND ENHANCEMENT TECHNOLOGY

**TYPE OF ASSISTIVE
LISTENING DEVICE**

LOOP	FM	INFRARED	HARDWIRE	DESIRABLE QUALITIES
N	Y	Y	Y	ACCESSIBLE
Y	N	N	Y	INEXPENSIVE
Y	N	N	Y	DURABLE
N	Y	N	N	MANY USES IN DIFFERENT SITUATIONS
N	N	Y	Y	FREE FROM INTERFERENCE
Y	N	N	N	EASY TO MONITOR
Y	N	N	Y	ALWAYS CHARGED
Y	Y	Y	N	YOU CAN SIT ANYWHERE
Y	N	N	N	FREE OF SANITARY PROBLEMS
Y	Y	Y	Y	SOUNDS OK TO OTHERS
Y	Y	N	N	ADJUSTS TO HEARING LOSS
N	Y	N	N	CAN BE USED OUTDOORS
Y	N	N	Y	SIMPLE TO OPERATE
N	Y	N	N	MULITPLE CONVERSATIONS
Y	N	N	N	REQUIRES A "T" SWITCH ON HEARING AID
N	Y	N	N	FUNCTIONS OVER LONG DISTANCES
N	N	N	Y	FREE FROM SILENT SPOTS
Y	N	N	Y	EASY REPAIRS
Y	N	N	Y	EASY TO TROUBLESHOOT
N	Y	N	N	EASY TO INSTALL
Y	N	N	N	GOOD COSMETICS

Y = YES   N = NO

Figure 5-4: Summary of Sound Enhancement Technology.

need only be placed within six inches of the TV or video speaker to provide a good S/N. In addition, many transmitters have the capability of being directly plugged into the speaker systems (audio-out plug) of TV or video equipment, given appropriate connecting cords. **It is important for college students with hearing loss to know that a significant amount of lecture material may be presented via video monitor.** Because the sound coming from video monitors may be of poor quality, it is crucial for college students who are hearing impaired to use some sort of sound enhancement technology.

Telecaption Decoders

The National Captioning Institute (NCI) was established in 1979 by the U.S. Department of Education to make television viewing accessible to persons with hearing loss (Vaughn & Lightfoot, 1987). Through the process of "closed captioning," narration, dialogue, and sound effects of TV programs are translated into captions which run across the bottom of the television screen. The captioning service is free, provided by TV, cable, and video industries with over one hundred ten hours of programming available each week. However, in order to receive the captions, one must purchase a "Telecaption II Adapter," for approximately $200. Without the Telecaption Adapter, the captions remain invisible. Many of the college students with hearing loss enjoy the captions, and interestingly, caption use has been linked to improvement in reading skills.

Telecommunication Technology

The ability to use the telephone is crucial for both business and social contacts. There are many types of amplifiers available which can allow telephone communication to be enjoyable, not stressful. Because of the numbers and variety of devices available, and because of individual needs, the reader is advised to actually try several amplifiers (at your speech and hearing center) before purchasing one.

Some amplifiers are portable, while some are built into the telephone handset. Some allow for variable amplification, while some amplify to a fixed amount. The typical amplified handset and portable strap-on amplifier provide approximately 30 percent amplification of the incoming voice (Vaughn & Lightfoot, 1987). Some amplifiers are hearing aid compatible, and some are not. Some people take off their hearing aids and use the amplified handset, some people keep their hearing aids on the "M" setting while using a telephone amplifier, and some people put their aids on the "T" setting while using the amplifier. Some people prefer a speakerphone where the voice from the phone is amplified into the room, avoiding the issue of appropriately positioning the phone next to the hearing aid. So you see, there are many options for telephone use. The cost for telephone amplifiers varies from about $18 to $250.

Have a "T" Switch on Your Hearing Aid

Making sure that you have a "T" switch on your hearing aid will provide for greater options and flexibility for telephone use, and for use of assistive communication devices in general. The "T" switch turns off the hearing aid microphone and activates the magnetic induction coil within the hearing aid (see Chapters 3 and 4). This coil will pick up signals from the magnetic field generated by certain telephones and telephone amplifiers. Because the hearing aid microphone is off, background noise is eliminated, allowing the listener to concentrate on the telephone conversation. In addition, using the "T" switch will eliminate the feedback often caused by trying to listen on the phone with the hearing aid in the "M" position. Unfortunately, many all-in-the-ear hearing aids are too small to allow a strong enough telecoil to be built-in. Therefore, the person might require ear-level hearing aids in order to accommodate an appropriate telecoil. In addition, when purchasing a telephone amplifier, make sure that it is hearing aid compatible; that it generates a magnetic field.

A person with a moderately-severe, severe, or profound hearing loss might need to make the following telephone accommodations (Centa, 1986): have a strong "T" coil built into the hearing aid; have a strong, hearing aid compatible amplifier; spend time learning how to most efficiently use this telephone equipment; develop additional telephone strategies.

Castle (1980) and Erber (1985) have suggested numerous techniques to enhance telephone communication. Simple steps, like repeating back information to the caller to make sure that it was understood, spelling names and hard-to-hear words, and making sure that the message was understood by both parties, can avoid later confusions.

Telecommunication Devices for Persons Who Are Deaf—TDD

Some individuals have hearing losses so profound that telephone word discrimination is not possible, even with telephone amplifiers. In these cases, a TDD would be very helpful, Figure 5-5. Based on the TTY (teletypewriter) idea of two typewriters talking by wire, the TDD also has letters appearing on a screen or printer (Cutler, 1986). About the

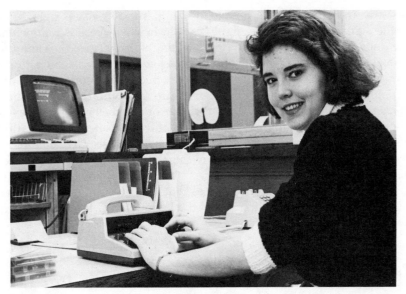

Figure 5-5: A TDD Allows a Typed Message to Be Sent Via Telephone to Another TDD.

size of a small typewriter, a TDD can communicate only with another TDD, requires power provided by either batteries or wall connection, and the message needs to be typed on the thirty-two-letter keyboard. Approximate cost varies from about $169 to $1700 depending upon size, model, and sophistication.

The 1982 Telecommunications for the Disabled Act included help for persons who are hearing impaired (Vaughn & Lightfoot, 1987). Specifically, certain telephones were regarded as "essential" and were designated to be hearing aid compatible, being equipped with a receiver that generates a magnetic field and having volume controls. These essential telephones included coin-operated telephones and those provided for emergency use in elevators, along highways, in tunnels and bridges. The FCC additionally stated that a portion of new telephones in hotel and motel rooms, hospitals, nursing homes, and public parts of offices and businesses be hearing aid compatible. **Telephones that have a blue connection to the handset cord are designed to work with the "T" switch on your hearing aid.**

Signal Alerting Technology

Any device which warns, signals, or alerts, is included in this category (Wayner, 1986). These devices can be hardwire or wireless systems and can provide very loud sound signals, visual signals, or tactile signals. For example, lights can flash when there is a knock at the door, when the telephone rings, when the baby cries, or when the smoke alarm goes off. A small vibrator attached to your wrist can perform the same task. Flashing lights can awaken one in the morning as can a vibrator placed under the pillow or mattress of the bed. Extra loud buzzers can be attached to the telephone or doorbell. There are even "hearing-ear" dogs who are trained to notify the person with hearing loss (by jumping on them to get their attention) of selective sounds in the environment. In short, if the environmental monitoring function of hearing (as mentioned in Chapter 2) is severely interrupted by the hearing loss, there are numerous devices that can substitute. Prices range from $20 to $600 depending upon the product and flexibility of the device.

Psycho-Social Issues

With all of the available communication devices, persons with hearing loss need only purchase the appropriate equipment in order to participate in societal interactions. Right?? Wrong!! Surprisingly, assistive communication devices account for less than 3 percent of the income of the hearing health care industry (Leavitt, 1987). Why are so few people actually taking advantage of the available equipment that can make life so much easier?

There are many issues surrounding the use of such equipment which must be considered (Leavitt, 1985, 1987), including visual deviance, experience with equipment use, emotional support, and practice. Simply explaining the advantages of such technology and then making the equipment available will not promote its use (Flexer, Wray, & Black, 1986; Leavitt, 1985, 1987).

The cost of using any assistive communication device is calling attention to oneself and one's hearing loss. Think about it. None of this technology is invisible. If it is not "OK" to have a hearing loss, then it is certainly not "OK" to advertise this loss (see Chapter 12). Students who are just beginning to attend the college support group often comment that they would rather flunk a course than ask the professor to wear even a small microphone. The value of the instrument cannot compete with the devalued feeling that students report experiencing as a result of announcing their hearing loss.

For instance, the same graduate student who named the FM unit "the clarifier" said that he was initially very embarrassed when the professor told the whole class that he was wearing the microphone (FM transmitter) because "that student over there has a hearing loss and needs this to hear better." While the professor meant well, the student said that he wished that he could crawl into a hole when everyone in the lecture hall turned to look at him. Because of support received in the college group, this student continues to use the equipment, but he admitted to having second thoughts. The point is, equipment use will not automatically occur. Technology needs to be supplemented by: successful users promoting the equipment; hands-on experience in sheltered situations; an improved group image (hearing loss is OK); and a group of friends who can provide emotional support through the initial stages of experimentation with technology (Flexer, Wray, Black, & Millin, 1987).

Summary

The purpose of this chapter has been to acquaint people with the large variety of readily available assistive communication devices. Through the use of technology, the college student with a hearing loss can gain access to social interactions that had previously been denied.

Equipment use is not a simple matter, however. Psycho-social issues must also be considered, and college students typically need support as they try new devices and become comfortable with managing their hearing losses.

National Distributors of Assistive Communication Devices

I. **National resources for information on devices in general:**
   A. New York League for the Hard of Hearing
      71 West 23rd Street, New York, NY 10010-4162
      212-741-7650/TTY—212-255-1932
      (They also have an excellent videotape demonstrating the use of various devices.)
   B. Self Help for Hard of Hearing People, Inc. (SHHH)
      7800 Wisconsin Ave., Bethesda, MD.   20814
      301-657-2248, Voice, or 301-657-2249, TTY
II. **Sound Enhancement Technology**
   A. Companies manufacturing FM equipment:
      1. Audio Enhancement (Comtek)
         #8 Winfield Pointe Lane, St. Louis, MO   63141
         314-567-6141

2. Earmark
    1125 Dixwell Ave., Hamden, CT   06514
    302-777-2130
3. Phonic Ear
    250 Camino Alto, Mill Valley, CA   94941
    414-383-4000 and 1-800-227-0735
4. Telex Communications
    9600 Aldrich Ave., S., Minneapolis, MN   55420
    1-800-328-8212
5. Williams Sound Corp.
    5929 Baker Rd., Minnetonka, MN 55345-5997
    612-931-0291

B. Induction Loop Systems
1. Oticon Corporation (Minicom Loop System)
    29 Schoolhouse Rd., P.O. Box 424,
    Somerset, NJ   08873
    201-560-1220 and 1-800-526-3921
2. Rastronics ALD's, N.J., HARC Mercantile
    3130 Portage St., P.O. 3055
    Kalamazoo, MI   49003-3055
    1-800-445-9968

C. Infrared Systems
1. Audex
    713 N. Fourth St., Longview, TX   75601
    214-758-9392 and 1-800-442-8489
2. Siemens Hearing Instruments
    10 Constitution Ave., P.O. Box 1397
    Piscataway, NJ   08855

D. Hardwire Systems
1. Most of the companies mentioned above also have hardwire units, e.g., Williams Sound.
2. Components from Radio Shack can also be put together to make a functional, inexpensive hardwire unit (Sudler & Flexer, 1986).
3. Eckstein Bros., Inc.
    4807 W. 118 Place, Hawthorne, CA 90250
    213-772-6113
4. Hear You Are, Inc.
    4 Musconetcong Ave., Stanhope, NJ   07874

III. **Television Enhancement Technology**
A. All of the above listed devices can also be used to improve television and radio listening.
B. Telecaption Decoding
    National Captioning Institute, Inc.
    Dept. DM, 5203 Leesburg Pike, 15th Floor
    Falls Church, VA   22041
    1-800-528-6600, Voice or 703-998-2400, Voice or TTY

IV. Telecommunication Technology (telephone amplifiers)

   A. AT&T Special Needs Center (for general information)
       2001 Route 46, Parsippany, NJ   07054
       1-800-233-1222 or 1-800-833-3232, TTY

   B. Allied Hearing, Dept. 54
       6545 France Ave., #614, Edina, MN 55435
       612-929-0501

   C. Hal-Hen
       35-53 24th St., P.O. Box 6077
       Long Island City, NY   11106
       718-392-6020

   D. HARC Mercantile
       P.O. Box 3055, Kalamazoo, MI   49003-3055
       1-800-445-9968

V. Telecommunication Devices for the Deaf—TDD

   A. Krown Research, Inc.
       10371 W. Jefferson Blvd., Culver City, CA   90232
       1-800-344-3277

   B. Phone—TTY
       202 Lexington Ave., Hackensack, NJ   07601
       Voice/TTY: 201-489-7889

   C. Ultratec, Inc.
       6442 Normandy Lane, Madison, WI   53719-1119
       1-800-482-2424 or Voice/TTD: 608-273-0707

VI. Signal Alerting Technology . . . Warning Devices

   A. Nationwide Flashing Signal Systems
       8120 Fenton St., Silver Spring, MD   20910

   B. Quest Electronics
       510 S. Worthington St., Oconomowoc, WI   53066
       1-800-558-9526

   C. Sonic Alert, Inc.
       1750 W. Hamlin Rd., Rochester Hills, MI   48309

Caution: The above list is not exhaustive, but was meant to acquaint the reader with a variety of equipment options. In addition, many companies carry several different types of technology. The consumer is encouraged to investigate closely many companies and products to find those most appropriate for his/her needs.

References

Berg, F.S. (1986). Classroom acoustics and signal transmission. In F.S. Berg, J.C. Blair, S.H. Viewheg, & A. Wilson-Vlotman (Eds.), *Educational Audiology for the Hard of Hearing Child* (pp. 157–180). Orlando, FL: Grune & Stratton.

Berg, F. (1987). *Facilitating Classroom Listening: A Handbook for Teachers of Normal and Hard-of-Hearing Students*. Boston: College Hill Press/Little, Brown Company.

Castle, D.L. (1980). *Telephone Training for the Deaf.* Rochester, NY: National Technical Institute for the Deaf.

Centa, J.M. (1986). Telephones can be helpful hearing aids. *SHHH, 8,* 9–11.

Cutler, B. (1986). Telephones and TDD's for hard of hearing people. *SHHH, 7,* 25–26.

Diedrichsen, R. (1987). Towards the acquisition of basic rights and services for persons who are hard of hearing. *SHHH, 8,* 3–4.

Erber, N.P. (1985). *Telephone Communication and Hearing Impairment.* San Diego, CA: College Hill Press.

Flexer, C., Wray, D.F., & Black, T.S., (1986). Support group for moderately hearing impaired college students: An expanding awareness. *The Volta Review, 88,* 223–229.

Flexer, C., Wray, D., Black, T., & Millin, J. (1987). Amplification devices: Evaluating classroom effectiveness for moderately hearing impaired college students. *The Volta Review, 89,* 347–357.

Leavitt, R.J. (1985). Counseling to encourage use of SNR enhancing systems. *Hearing Instruments, 36,* 8–9.

Leavitt, R.J. (1987). Promoting the use of rehabilitation technology. *ASHA, 29,* 28–31.

Leavitt, R.J., & Hodgson, W.R. (1984). An effective home FM induction loop system. *Hearing Instruments, 35,* 14–15; 47.

Ross, M. (1986). Thoughts on ALD's. *Hearing Instruments, 37,* 16–21.

Smith, C.F. (1985). Induction loop systems. *Hearing Instruments, 36,* 26.

Sudler, W.H., & Flexer, C. (1986). Low-cost assistive listening device. *Language, Speech and Hearing Services in Schools, 17,* 342–344.

Vaughn, G.R. (1986). Bill of rights for listeners and talkers. *Hearing Instruments, 37,* 8.

Vaughn, G.R., & Lightfoot, R.K. (1987). ALD's pioneers: Past and present. *Hearing Instruments, 38,* 4–6; 9–12.

Vaughn, G.R., Lightfoot, R.K., & Gibbs, S.D. (1983). Assistive listening devices . . . Part III: Space. *ASHA, 25,* 33–46.

Wayner, D.S. (1986). Assistive listening devices for improved communication and greater independence. *Hearing Instruments, 37,* 21–24.

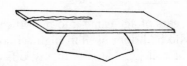

Chapter 6
Front-Row Seating Is Not Enough for Classroom Listening

James C. Blair, Ph.D.

Listening Problems

It has been found that most individuals with hearing impairments do not know what they can do to improve their own listening abilities (Berg, Blair, Viehweg, Wilson-Vlotman, 1986). It has also been reported that the vast majority of school administrators and teachers do not understand the importance of controlling noise and reverberation (echoes) in rooms in which these individuals are expected to be able to listen (Berg, 1987). Ross (1982) expressed the viewpoint that when all the other aspects of hearing have been carefully controlled, the individual with a hearing loss is unfortunately placed in an acoustic environment (a typical, noisy room) which is so poor that the person with the hearing loss has little or no chance for success.

The purpose of this chapter is to help the reader understand that listening is more than a passive activity for the person with a hearing impairment; improving the listening environment for these individuals is critical if they are going to reach their potential. In order to illustrate the problems that a person with a hearing loss encounters, the story of one young man is used as an illustrative device. We will trace his experience with listening through a variety of adventures in order to highlight the difficulties that similar students face on a daily basis, and also to illustrate some ways in which these difficulties might be reduced.

A Student with a Hearing Impairment

A young man of about eighteen years of age came into my office. He was a good looking young man, who had done well in high school and who was in his second quarter of college. He was in my office because the Office of Handicapped Services (see Chapter 8) had referred him to me. He had not performed well in his first quarter of school and the Office of Handicapped Services thought that perhaps my working with this young man might be of some help. As he spoke, he had a slight distortion of speech, omitting final /s/ sounds and other final sounds such as /t/ and /d/. However, I understood all that he said to me and he seemed to understand all that I said to him. He wore two behind-the-ear hearing aids, which were barely noticeable because his hair was worn fairly long and covered his ears slightly.

I asked him why he felt that he had not done well in his school work. He indicated that the professors tended to talk too fast, and that they asked questions on the examinations that were not in the readings. I asked if he had difficulty understanding what the teachers said. He said that he did not think so; he may have missed some of the information, but he did not feel that it was a significant amount.

We tested his hearing and found that without his hearing aids he could not understand conversational speech, since he had a 75 dB hearing loss in his left ear and a 65 dB loss in his right ear. With his hearing aids on, his hearing improved into the mild loss range, and his ability to understand conversational speech while wearing his hearing aids was 95 percent in the right ear, and 90 percent in the left, using word lists that were quite difficult (for example the word *laud* is one of the choices). However, when we tested his ability to understand speech in a background of noise, he experienced considerable difficulty understanding speech. His discrimination score fell to 50 percent when noise (i.e., eight talkers talking at the same time in one speaker, and one talker, the one the subject was to listen to, from the other speaker) was presented at a level where the speech was 6 dB louder than the noise. The testing was done in this way because we have found that the relationship between the noise and speech in average college and high school classrooms is about +6 dB (where speech is louder than the noise). Thus, when the environment was similar to the one in which he had to listen in a typical classroom, his ability to understand speech was greatly affected. We tested him a little further and found that when he was able to see the talker and to hear in a background of noise, his scores improved to 98 percent. This suggests that his ability to cope when he could both see and hear the talker, even in a background of noise, was excellent.

I spoke with him about these results and asked him some questions about where he seated himself in the classroom, and the problems that he felt he had listening in noise. He indicated that he noticed if he was not able to see the speaker clearly, he was not able to understand as well. He additionally indicated that he usually came to class a little late and would end up sitting near the back of the room. I asked him if it was more difficult when he sat near the rear. He said that he was not sure.

The Inverse Square Law or the Distance Effect

I explained that there were a couple of things that might make it difficult for him to understand the speech of the professor while seated at the rear. First, there is a law called the inverse square law. According to this law the sound pressure (or our perception of intensity) decreases by 6 dB when the distance between the speaker and the receiver is doubled.

I also explained that frequency, the second major dimension of sound, is the number of times the sound wave vibrates in one second. If we cannot hear all frequencies well, we misunderstand what people say. The term used to describe frequency is cycles per second (cps), or Hertz (Hz). The higher the number of vibrations which occur in one second, the higher our perception of pitch. Table 6-1 illustrates some of the more common environmental sounds and their intensity and frequencies.

As suggested earlier, the inverse square law says that the further away from the sound one is, the softer the amount of pressure that is exerted on the eardrum, and the less intense the sound. Figure 6-1 illustrates this principle. Notice that the person sitting sixteen feet from the speaker hears at a level which is 24 dB softer than it was only one foot from the speaker's mouth.

Of course, the inverse square law is most accurate in an area with totally sound absorbent walls and a width which is infinite. In an enclosed classroom, the inverse square law is not a completely accurate predictor of the way that sounds work. However, it is clear that as distance increases, there is a significant reduction in the intensity level of the signal. The actual effect on listening has been studied by a number of researchers (Bess & McConnell, 1981; Berg, Blair, Viehweg, & Watkins, 1983). One of the research findings in college classrooms has been that all rooms have a degree of background noise in them and that the level of the teacher's voice in the classroom is often softer than the level

TABLE 6-1. THE INTENSITY AND FREQUENCY LEVELS OF SOME COMMON ENVIRONMENTAL SOUNDS.

Intensity Levels (dB HL)	Frequency Area (Hertz)	Environmental Sounds
100–110	Low (125–250)	Powered Lawnmower
110–120	Mid (500–2000)	Rock Band
110–120	High (3000–8000)	Jet Airplane
80–90	Low (250–500)	Street Noise Barking Dog
80–90	Mid (500–2000)	Telephone (3 feet)
60–70	Low (125–250)	Window Airconditioner (High Level)
60–70	Mid (500–2000)	Baby Crying
60–70	High (3000–8000)	Singing Birds
40–50	Mid (500–4000)	Soft Speech
20–30	Low (125–350)	Bedroom at Night
0–10	Mid (1000–2000)	Wind Blowing Gently Through Bushes

of the noise! It has been found, for example, that the noise in classrooms is about 56 dB SPL, and the average level of the teachers voice at the front of the room is about 65 dB SPL. By the time the speech reaches the back of the room, the speech intensity will have decreased to about 50 dB, while the noise will remain at the same level. Thus at the back of the room, the speech has been measured to be about 6 dB softer than the noise. The effect on listening, in this kind of environment, is profound, especially for individuals with hearing loss. We found that when we expected college students to write simple sentences in a very quiet environment at a short distance (six feet) from the speaker, they wrote

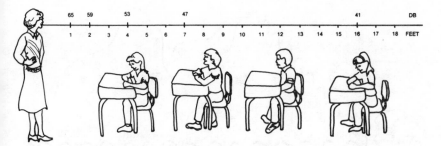

Figure 6-1: The Effects of Distance on the Intensity of a Signal.

the sentences accurately 95 percent of the time. However, when we asked them to do the equivalent activity in a classroom which was noisy (speech slightly louder than the noise), they were accurate only 50 percent of the time.

The implications are that the average student with a hearing loss sitting in a regular classroom will experience great difficulty understanding even simple speech. Often these students will try to compensate by watching the speaker's lips, but even under these circumstances, the student will typically do less well than one might think.

Reverberation or the Echo Effect

If the factors of noise and distance were our only concern, we might be able to overcome the problem. However, there is an additional factor that will usually create listening difficulties for persons with hearing impairments. This factor is reverberation time. Reverberation is the amount of reflected sound there is in a room. Figure 6-2 illustrates how sound is transmitted from the speaker in direct waves, and how these direct waves literally bounce off of hard surfaces to send second, or even third waves of sound back into the room. Reverberation is measured in time, and is defined in terms of the amount of time it takes for a sound, once it has stopped being produced, to decrease in intensity 60 dB. When reverberation times are long (it takes a long time for echoes to stop once sound is produced), listeners have a more difficult time understanding speech. The overall affect is that there is a slurring or blending of the sounds together so that the individual sounds become unclear.

Individuals with normal hearing can tolerate reverberation times up to one second with minimal effects on discrimination. However, once the reverberation exceeds one second, even those of us with normal hearing begin to experience some problems. The reverberation in a gym-

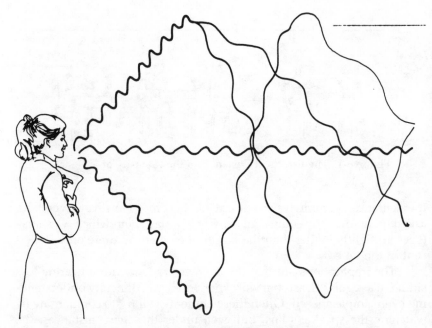

Figure 6-2: Reverberation is the Length of Time it Takes for a Sound to Stop Vibrating Once It Has Stopped. The Heavy Lines Represent the Original Sound and the Lighter Lines Represent the Reflected Sound.

nasium is about one and one-half seconds, and most people have some problems understanding speech in this setting. Individuals with hearing impairments experience difficulties understanding speech at even shorter reverberation times than normal hearers. For example, the individual with normal hearing will be able to repeat back words at nearly 100 percent accuracy until the reverberation time is above one second, but the individual with a hearing loss will start having trouble repeating words when the reverberation time is only about 0.5 seconds. We are not sure why the person with a hearing loss experiences difficulty at lower reverberation times. It seems that these individuals need all their abilities to understand speech under the best of circumstances, and when there are extraneous variables added to their already faulty auditory systems, their abilities to use their hearing are significantly reduced.

Thus, in order for individuals with hearing impairment to use their auditory skills to the maximum possible level, it is very important that the distance from the speaker, the amount of noise in the room, and the level of reverberation, all be taken into consideration. Unfortunately, these factors are typically overlooked when individuals with hearing loss are integrated into regular classrooms.

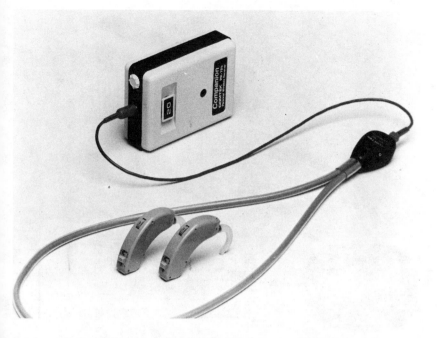

Figure 6-3: Inductance Neck Loop with the Switch on Hearing Aid Set to
Both the Microphone (M) and Telecoil (T). (Used with permission of
COMTEK, Salt Lake City, Utah)

Solutions to the Problem

We shared the information we collected with the young man with
the hearing loss who was introduced at the beginning of the chapter.
Given the information about the classroom situation and the way that
he seated himself in those rooms, it was suggested that he try a few
things. First, he should try to seat himself in the second row of the class,
a little to one side of the professor's usual lecturing position. Second, I
suggested that he should try using an FM system during the lectures,
to see if this piece of equipment might be useful in helping him improve
his classroom performance.

He indicated that he would do the first thing, but the second
suggestion he really had no experience with and did not know how to
respond. I explained that an FM system came in a variety of forms (see
Figures 6-3 and 6-4). For example, he could plug the FM receiver into
his personal hearing aids, or he could wear a neck loop (see Figure
6-3) which would mean he would need to wear his hearing aid on the
telecoil setting, or he could take his hearing aids off and wear the FM

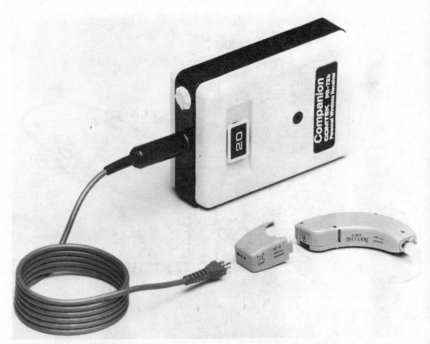

Figure 6-4: Earlevel Hearing Aid Acoustic (Shoe) Coupling and a Wire Which Attaches to the FM Receiver. (Used with permission of COMTEK, Salt Lake City, Utah).

receiver amplifier in conjunction with an insert receiver that could be placed in his ear directly.

Problems with the Solutions

As he examined these pieces of equipment, he appeared resistant and stated that he was not willing to try them at all. I asked him why. He indicated that the FM unit was so large that all the people in class would immediately know that he had a hearing impairment, and thus he would not be accepted by the class. The second reason he did not like to use the FM was that he would have to talk directly to the professors and would be expecting them to wear a broadcasting microphone. He was not sure that he had the courage to do this. I asked if he would be willing to participate in some experiences to determine if an FM system would make any difference. He indicated that he was reasonable and that he would be willing to try some things.

TABLE 6-2. COMPARATIVE LISTENING PERCENTAGES OF 7 COLLEGE-AGE STUDENTS WHO WERE HEARING IMPAIRED USING HEARING AIDS VERSUS VARIOUS OTHER FORMS OF AMPLIFICATION IN 2 ROOMS WITH DIFFERENT REVERBERATION TIMES (RT).

Description of Amplification	Room A .5 RT	Room B 1.67 RT
Personal Hearing Aid	75%	36%
FM Receiver with Direct Wire to Button Receiver	80%	78%
Personalized FM with Inductive (Neck Loop) Coupling		
Brand I	DNT	18%
Brand II	78%	85%
Brand III	75%	78%
Public Address System	90%	48%

Does FM Really Work in the Classroom?

In order to determine if FM systems would be of any value in college classrooms, we developed three experiences.

Experience 1:

Seven students with hearing losses in the mild to moderately severe range (the average hearing loss was 48 dB) were tested. These seven subjects scored an average of 88 percent on word discrimination lists, suggesting that all of these subjects had excellent potential for using their hearing as a primary means for learning.

Simple sentences were read to the students, and they were asked to write their responses while they were in two classrooms under different conditions (see Table 6-2). The best possible listening scores were obtained when the student wore an FM system. However, it was also clear that the type of classroom the person was in made a large difference. If the person was going to wear a hearing aid and refused to use an FM or other assistive device, it was very important that the person be in a room that was quiet during the times when a talker was trying to communicate something of value, and that reverberation times be low.

Experience 2:

We next tested the college students in different reverberant environments and found that the reduction of reverberation helped the subjects with hearing loss improve their ability to understand speech (Berg, Blair, Viehweg & Watkins, 1983). A study completed by Finitzo-Hieber and Tillman (1978) supports the conclusion that we reached, that a significant reduction in reverberation and noise in a classroom can improve the discrimination ability of individuals with hearing impairments. In fact, even minor changes in noise and/or reverberation will begin to affect the ability of students with hearing loss to do better in school.

Classroom Amplification Systems

Another type of amplification system that was successfully used with children with mild hearing losses, was described by Sarff (1981). This classroom amplification system consists of a teacher microphone, an FM transmitter, and an FM receiver amplifier. In addition one or more speakers are placed either in the ceiling or in front or in back of the classroom so as to be above the heads of the listeners, but facing at an angle pointing toward the chairs.

As we read this study, a question arose whether sound field FM would be of value for youngsters with moderate hearing loss. This kind of questioning led us to try another kind of experience with the college students with the hearing losses. By this time, however, our original group of college students were a little weary of our constant questions. We thus decided that we would set up the third experience for a different group of students who were hearing impaired, but that we would discuss the results with our college students.

Experience 3:

We were able to locate ten students who demonstrated mild to moderate sensorineural hearing loss. We went to a regular school classroom in order to make the data we collected as realistic as possible. We decided that we would try three different types of amplification: (1) the students' personal hearing aids, (2) an FM sound field system, and (3) an FM neck loop system which was used in conjunction with the students' personal hearing aids (see Blair, Myrup and Viehweg, 1989, for a complete description).

We discovered that sound field FM could be a useful tool for individuals with moderate hearing losses while wearing their hearing aids.

We also found, however, that the best possible scores are obtained when using a personal FM, such as the one depicted in Figures 6-3 and 6-4.

Summary of Experiences

At the conclusion of all these experiences, we again talked with our college students with hearing impairments about what we were able to discover. It appeared that no matter what we did, the conclusions became more obvious. A hearing aid, although very important for the basic survival of a person with a hearing loss, is not a very good tool to use in a learning situation, when compared to any kind of working FM system. The use of the FM sound field system was of significant value to the hearing impaired in a regular classroom. It was also clear that the best possible advantages came to persons with hearing loss when they wore a personal FM system.

Other Considerations

In the discussion above, we focused on the ability of the individual with a hearing loss to use his/her hearing to facilitate learning in a variety of educational environments. We have not discussed the importance of the visual system as an aid to the individual with hearing loss in a communication exchange. However, it is clear, in most cases, that the visual sense is an additional factor which assists the individual with a hearing loss in understanding what people say.

Research (Sanders, 1982; Montgomery, Walden & Prosek, 1987) has suggested that the benefits derived from the visual sense are not, on the average, as good as we would like. Frequently, because of the nature of the speaker, the environment, or the message, the person who is dependent on the visual system is unable to use the visual sense as a reliable tool for receiving information.

Therefore, even a good speechreader will have a great deal of difficulty understanding the teacher in a typical instructional situation if the student is not able to use the auditory sense to the highest extent possible. Based on our observations, the average student with a hearing loss with good speechreading ability would likely understand merely 20 percent of a message through lipreading alone. The same individual in a typical classroom environment, wearing a good hearing aid (but no FM system) and able to see the teacher all the time, will understand less than 50 percent of the message.

Conclusion

Recall that, at the beginning of this chapter, a young man with a hearing loss who was eighteen years old was described. After we had collected the data reported above, we met once again with this young man to discuss the findings. As we looked at his individual scores in all of the conditions, he could see that he did considerably better when using a personal FM system. He agreed that the best thing he could do for himself was to try an FM system for one quarter, and thus determine for himself if it would improve his ability to function.

He took the FM system and used it consistently during that quarter. He also came to see me once a week to report on his successes and failures. It became very clear to him, as he used the equipment, that it was of tremendous value. He encountered no problem in getting the professors to use the equipment. At the end of the quarter, his grades in every subject area were significantly better.

Our experience has been that, in most instances, when college students with hearing loss begin to use the FM systems on a regular basis, they will typically be able to function at a higher level than they do when they do not use the systems. We have also found that when the FM systems are used properly, the students become advocates of their use with other students, and cannot understand why a peer with a hearing loss would not give the system a try.

The important thing to remember is that listening is not simply a matter of trying harder, or even sitting in the best place in the room. Most individuals with hearing loss need to have the advantages that they can obtain from the use of a personal FM system.

Checklist of an Optimal Classroom Environment

1. Acoustical characteristics:
   a. Background noise:
      _____ Very poor conditions (normal listeners have difficulty understanding speech).
      _____ Poor conditions (normal listeners have occasional difficulty understanding speech).
      _____ Good conditions (normal listeners can easily understand what is said without difficulty).
      _____ Excellent conditions (the speaker's voice is significantly louder than any noise that might be present [amplified]).
   b. Acoustical treatment of the room:

_____ Minimal acoustical treatment in the room (hard plaster walls, no carpet on the floor, wooden or hard surface on the ceiling).

_____ Partial treatment of the room (carpet on the floor, and acoustic tile on the ceiling).

_____ Full acoustic treatment (carpet on the floor, drapes over the windows, acoustic tile on the ceiling, no more than one wall without some sort of absorbent material covering the wall, and solid core doors)

2. Amplification systems:

_____ All students with hearing loss wear their hearing aids and the hearing aids are in good working order.

_____ Students have access to assistive devices that are compatible with the needs of the students.

_____ The classroom or other learning environment is equipped with sound field equipment that is used by the instructor.

3. Visual characteristics:

a. Teacher's face:

_____ Teacher's face is not clearly visible.

_____ Teacher's face is occasionally not clearly visible.

_____ There is no distraction from the teacher's face.

b. Control of the visual environment:

_____ Room too dark or lights insufficient for comfortable vision.

_____ Comfortable lighting for ease of working.

c. Window light is used to provide optimal illumination on working surfaces and on the teacher's face for speechreading:

_____ Students are facing the window(s) with the teacher's back to the window(s).

_____ Students and teacher with one side toward the window(s).

_____ Students with back to the window(s) and the teacher facing the window(s).

d. Seating arrangement:

_____ Some students cannot see either the teacher or other students from their regular seat.

_____ All the students can see the teacher, but some cannot see each other.

_____ All the students can see the teacher and one another from their regular seats.

References

Berg, F. (1987). *Facilitating Classroom Listening*. Boston: College Hill Press.

Berg, F., Blair, J., Viehweg, S., & Watkins, S. (1983). Listening in classrooms, hard-of-hearing. Final report, Regional Education Programs for Deaf and

Other Handicapped Persons (Postsecondary). Grant No. 600810357, U.S. Department of Education. Logan: Utah State University.

Berg, F., Blair, J., Viehweg, S., & Wilson-Vlotman, A. (1986). *Educational Audiology for the Hard of Hearing Child*. Orlando, FL: Grune & Stratton.

Bess, F., McConnell, F. (1981). *Audiology, Education and the Hearing Impaired Child*. St. Louis: C. V. Mosby Co.

Blair, J., Myrup, C., Viehweg, S. (1989). Comparison of the listening effectiveness of hard-of-hearing children using three types of amplification. *Educational Audiology Monograph.*, 1, pp. 48–55.

Finitzo-Hieber, T., & Tillman, T. (1978). Room acoustics effects on monosyllabic word discrimination ability of normal and hearing impaired children. *Journal of Speech & Hearing Research, 21*, 440–458.

Montgomery, A., Walden, B., & Prosek, R. (1987). Effects of consonantal context on vowel lipreading. *Journal of Speech & Hearing Research, 30*, 59–59.

Ross, M., with Brackett, D., Maxon, A. (1982). *Hard-of-Hearing Children in Regular Schools*. Englewood Cliffs: Prentice Hall.

Sanders, D. (1982). *Aural Rehabilitation*. Englewood Cliffs: Prentice Hall.

Sarff, L. (1981). An innovative use of free field amplification in regular classroom. In Roeser, R., & Downs, M. *Auditory Disorders in School Children*. New York: Thieme-Stratton.

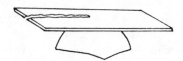

Chapter 7
Vocational Rehabilitation Services for College Students Who are Hearing Impaired

George Kosovich, M.A., M.Ed.

When I started writing this chapter I found myself thinking about my early college career. I flunked out of college twice! While there were a number of reasons for this poor performance, my inability to do college level work was not one of them. The fact that I have since earned two masters degrees is proof of my academic abilities.

Although I had a significant hearing loss in my early college days, my hearing impairment did not create my college failure. In fact I later earned two masters degrees after losing a lot more hearing.

One thing that did help me succeed in college was the assistance that I got from my state's vocational rehabilitation agency. Apparently these valuable vocational rehabilitation services made quite an impression on me, because when I graduated from college I started working for the state vocational rehabilitation agency with people who were hearing impaired. I liked working with this group because I felt that I had an understanding of what college students with hearing losses have to cope with. I know how expensive college can be. I understand the frustrations of struggling to hear in a large classroom. I understand how exhausting it can be to try to take notes and lipread the teacher at the same time. I know the frustration of trying to communicate at a college dance when there is a lot of background noise. I understand how difficult it can be to try to lipread a person on television in a large classroom.

Fortunately, the state's vocational rehabilitation (VR) agency can help with many of these problems. For example, the VR agency can provide financial assistance for college tuition and books. The VR agency may be able to purchase hearing aids and the other technologies described in Chapter 5. The VR counselor can help you find a job. Those are some of the reasons why I enjoyed working as a VR counselor for so many years. That is also why I am glad to tell you what the vocational rehabilitation agency can do for you as you start college. I feel this information can make your college success much easier. So let's get to it, and learn about this valuable agency.

What Is Vocational Rehabilitation?

Vocational rehabilitation services in this country were started after World War I to help men who were disabled during the war to become productive citizens again. Since then, the VR program has expanded to provide job training for men and women of all disability groups. Today VR provides services to people who were born with a disability or who acquired a disability later in life. As a student with hearing impairment, you may be eligible for VR services whether you were born with a hearing loss or acquired it some time later.

Every state has a VR agency which is 80 percent funded by federal government money. The Rehabilitation Services Administration of the Department of Education oversees all state-operated VR agencies to assure that they are following federal rules and regulations. Consequently, VR agency rules and practices are similar from one state to another. However the way these services are provided can vary from state to state and even from city to city.

In general, VR services are designed to help people with disabilities get or keep a job in line with their abilities. Before you can receive any VR assistance you must demonstrate several things to your VR counselor.

First, you must show that your hearing loss causes a communication difficulty for you, especially in a classroom-type listening environment. A hearing and hearing aid evaluation from a certified audiologist can demonstrate this communication difficulty.

Second, you must show that your hearing loss is preventing you from getting the job you want. You must also show that this job requires some specialized college training.

Third, you must show that you can succeed in college classes required for your chosen profession. This test of your ability is usually based on your high-school performance and testing that is done by your VR counselor.

VR counselors want to get you into an occupation that meets your financial and intellectual needs. VR counselors are not just interested in helping you find a job. They are interested in helping you reach your employment potential! That is the good news about VR. So now all we need to do is teach you how to fit into the VR system. Hopefully, the information provided in the next few pages will show you how.

Making Yourself Eligible for VR Services

The first thing that will help you fit into the VR process is to understand that the services you receive from your VR agency are influenced by the relationship you have with your VR counselor. Having been a VR counselor for over ten years, I can assure you that it is much easier to provide services to someone who is reliable and hard working. If you are late for appointments, your VR counselor may wonder if you will not do the same thing when you become employed. Since every VR counselor has a large caseload, appointment tardiness also wastes a lot of other students' time.

Further, you must understand that your success in college reflects on your VR counselor's job performance since each VR counselor is required to show that a lot of clients have been rehabilitated each year. If you do poorly in college after VR has spent thousands of dollars for your education, it not only hurts your job prospects, but it affects your VR counselor's standing in the agency.

Here is a summary of ideas for developing a good working relationship with your VR counselor:

1. Do not be late or miss scheduled appointments with your VR counselor or other professional consultants.
2. Pay attention to your personal appearance when you visit your counselor. View each appointment as the early stage of a job interview. Dress professionally.
3. Recognize that money is limited in any VR agency. Take a full course load each term, and do well in school so that you do not have to repeat classes. Make an effort to carry as much of the financial load for college as you can. Seek other forms of financial aid, such as scholarships, work-study programs, parental support, and part-time jobs to help offset the high cost of your education.

If you follow the advice given above, your counselor will see that you are a reliable and hard-working student. This recognition will foster a good relationship and may even result in your counselor making a little extra effort to see that you are successful in college and in your later job-hunting activities.

The next thing that will help you fit into the VR system is to learn about your legal rights in the system. You must learn to stand up for these rights. All VR agencies receive federal money. As a result they cannot deny services to anyone on the basis of race, religion, sex, ethnic or national origin, age, residency, financial status, social membership, political preferences, or disability. If you are deaf and there are no counselors in your state who can communicate in sign language, you have the right to request a professional interpreter who is skilled in oral or signed interpretation. If you need a sound enhancement system to communicate in a group meeting with your VR counselor, you have the right to request such a system.

VR clients have the right to participate in the planning and provision of all rehabilitation services. This means that you help determine what services you will receive. Your VR counselor cannot decide which services you will receive without your input. You and your counselor must work together and agree on what is best for your college career.

As a VR client, you have the right to have all forms and papers explained to you in a language that you understand. Every VR agency uses a number of forms in the rehabilitation process. Some are more difficult to understand than others. If you do not understand the purpose of a form or letter, ask your VR counselor for an explanation. If necessary, your counselor will be available to help you complete financial aid forms, job applications, or any other forms directly related to your rehabilitation program. While it is important that you learn to do as much for yourself as possible, you should not be afraid to ask for assistance when necessary.

You should know that not every student with hearing impairment receives financial assistance from VR. Generally speaking, VR counselors want to serve students who are severely disabled, yet still have the potential to become successfully employed. According to VR regulations, a student is considered severely disabled if the average hearing loss in the better ear is 55 decibels or more at the frequencies of 500, 1000, and 2000 Hz. If your hearing loss is less than this, or if you do not see your hearing loss as a disability to your employment, you have less chance of receiving financial assistance from VR.

Another issue that you may need to address when considering eligibility for VR services is that of residency. Residency refers to the location of your "real" home. If you plan to go to college in another state, you may apply for VR services in that state. However, some VR counselors may be reluctant to serve you, particularly if you plan to return to your home state after college. Thus you should discuss the residency issue with the VR counselor in your state. Then decide in which state you will apply for VR services. You cannot be a VR client in two states at the same time, and your VR counselor will check to see that you are not receiving services in another state when you make your VR application.

The considerations discussed above will give you some insight into how you can fit into the VR process, and will increase your chances of receiving VR funding for your college career. Now we will look at how VR provides services to all potential clients and discuss the process as it relates to college students who are hearing impaired.

The Vocational Rehabilitation Process

Every state's VR agency uses a numbering system called the status system. This system, which is summarized below, helps a VR counselor keep track of where each client is in the rehabilitation process from the first day the client applies for services to the day the client is employed.

1. **Referral (Status 00).** This status acknowledges that a potential client has been referred to VR, and has provided basic identifying information to the VR counselor. This information includes name, address, social security number, and type of disability. At this point no decision has been made about eligibility for VR services.

2. **Application (Status 02).** A potential VR client is placed in Status 02 after completing the application form for VR services. When a potential client is placed in this status it usually means that the VR counselor has reason to believe this person is eligible for VR services. In this status, some money can be spent by VR for client evaluation, training, travel expenses, and hearing aids.

3. **Extended Evaluation (Status 06).** A person is placed in this status when it has been determined that a substantial handicap to employment exists, but the VR counselor is not sure that the client has the potential to benefit from VR services. A potential client will remain in this status until the VR counselor can gather enough information to determine whether VR services will be helpful. Since a determination of client eligibility can usually be made quickly, this status is not used very often.

4. **Closed As Ineligible from Status 00, 02 or 06 (Status 08).** When the VR counselor determines that an applicant does not meet one

of the eligibility requirements for VR service, that person is placed in Status 08. A person who has been receiving VR services may also be placed in this status when he or she moves away from the VR counselor's area and is no longer eligible for services.

5. **Certified Eligible (Status 10).** The applicant is certified eligible for VR services and placed in Status 10 when the counselor determines that the client meets the three eligibility requirements discussed previously.

    After eligibility for VR services has been established, the applicant and counselor must develop a written plan of action for achieving appropriate vocational goals. The next three status categories are used to classify the applicant while he or she is achieving these vocational goals.

6. **Counseling, Guidance and Placement Plan (Status 14).** In this status, the VR client is ready to be placed in a job and no further training or restoration services (as described below) are needed.

7. **Physical and Mental Restoration Plan (Status 16).** The VR client may be placed in this status when medical, psychiatric, or therapeutic services are required to help achieve vocational goals.

8. **Training (Status 18).** The primary service in Status 18 is education or on-the-job training. Most college students receiving financial assistance from VR will be in this status until graduation.

9. **Ready for Employment (Status 20).** A VR client who is ready for employment is occasionally placed here when training in Status 18 has been completed. However, this status is not often used since many clients get a job while still in Status 18.

10. **Employed (Status 22).** A VR client who is employed in what appears to be a permanent job will initially be placed in this status. After sixty days on this job, the client will often be moved to Status 26 which is described below.

11. **Services Interrupted (Status 24).** This status is used when a client in one of the status categories from 14 to 22 cannot continue in planned rehabilitation activities for any reason. This classification is often used rather than closing the client's file as unsuccessful.

12. **Closed Rehabilitated (Status 26).** This is every VR counselor's favorite status. When the client has been employed for 60 days and no further services are needed to maintain employment, the client's file can be closed. Every state VR agency measures its success by the number of people that achieve Status 26.

13. **Closed—Not Rehabilitated after Plan Services (Status 28).** This is every VR counselor's least favorite number. VR services have

been provided, but it does not appear that the client is capable of achieving any vocational goal. This status is also assigned to VR clients who cannot be located.

14. **Closed—Not Rehabilitated before Plan Services (Status 30).** This status is only used when a client has been declared eligible but does not go into a rehabilitation plan. For example, a client may be assigned to this status when he or she does not go into a rehabilitation plan such as Status 18 due to illness or relocation to another state.

15. **Post-Employment Services (Status 32).** This status is used for clients who were successfully employed, but now require additional VR services to maintain their present job or to find new employment.

16. **Closure Post-Employment Services (Status 33).** A client is assigned to Status 33 when VR services are no longer needed or when VR services will not make the client employable in the future.

Now let us see how this status system applies to a college student with a hearing impairment who is interested in receiving services from VR.

The Vocational Rehabilitation Process for Students with Hearing Impairment

Referral

Anyone can refer a student with hearing impairment to the state VR agency. A student can also go to VR without any referral. Typically, however, referrals are made by physicians that specialize in diseases of the ear, by audiologists, by school counselors, by Social Security Administration staff, or by employment service staff members.

Regardless of how you get to the agency, upon arrival, ask to be assigned to a VR counselor who has received specialized training in the area of hearing impairment. Such counselors are known as rehabilitation counselors for the deaf or RCDs. These counselors are usually fluent in sign language and have some training or work experience in the field of deafness. Unfortunately, experience has shown that RCDs typically have little experience working with people who are hard-of-hearing.

However, their knowledge of hearing loss, hearing aids, and other related issues is usually greater than the general VR counselor who serves all disability groups.

If there is no RCD available in your area, ask if there is a VR counselor in that office with previous experience working with people who are hearing impaired.

After your first contact with the VR agency, you will receive an appointment letter that will specify a time for you to meet with your counselor. At times this first meeting may be a group session, where the VR counselor explains VR rules and procedures to a group of potential clients. If your first meeting is in a group, you may request a loop or FM system. Alternatively, you might ask for a one-to-one meeting with your counselor. Both requests are within your rights as a person who is hearing impaired.

Before the first meeting with your counselor, you should do some planning. Develop some ideas about what services you would like to receive from VR. If you have had a hearing aid evaluation in the past year, you should bring this with you. You should have some ideas about hearing aids (see Chapter 4) and other technology (see Chapter 5) that you will need for college. You should have some ideas about occupations that are of interest to you (See Chapter 14 for ideas on how to choose potentially interesting occupations.) You should also have some ideas about which colleges provide training in your chosen occupations. Ideally, these colleges will also have loop or FM systems, notetakers, telecaption decoders, and amplified telephones available for students as required by federal regulations (Architectural and Transportation Barriers Compliance Board, 1982; Department of Health, Education and Welfare, 1977). Check with disabled student services at each college to determine if this technology is available.

Having all of this information available on your first visit to the VR counselor will show that you are organized and have started vocational planning. Such actions will favorably impress your counselor. Additionally, when you know what services you want, you are less dependent on someone else to make important choices for you. Since all VR counselors are not knowledgeable about the needs of students with hearing impairment, it is in your best interest to be prepared for this meeting. Do not be surprised if you need to explain FM and loop systems and other technology to your VR counselor. If you have a good working relationship, both of you will benefit from this discussion. Your VR counselor will become more aware of the needs of students who are hard-of-hearing and you might get VR funding for some of the technology that your chosen college does not currently provide.

Evaluation

Your VR counselor begins evaluating your potential as a client the first time you meet. However, the formal evaluation process does not begin until you have signed the VR application form.

The formal evaluation serves two purposes. First, the evaluation helps your counselor determine if you are eligible for services. Second, the evaluation helps determine what services are needed for you to finish college and become successfully employed.

For the average student who is hearing impaired, the average evaluation period is between one and two months. This extended period of time is necessary because a lot of academic and vocational testing must be completed to show that you have the ability to do college-level work.

During the formal evaluation period, three things must be established before you become eligible for VR assistance.

First, it must be established that you have a significant hearing loss.

Second, it must be shown that your hearing loss prevents you from getting or keeping a job you could otherwise perform.

Third, your VR counselor must be reasonably certain that you are capable of benefiting from college training and will become successfully employed after graduation.

Let us discuss how you can improve your chances of meeting these three requirements.

1. Proof of significant hearing loss

If you have not had a hearing and hearing aid evaluation in the past year, your VR counselor will pay to have this testing completed by a certified audiologist who is usually selected by your VR counselor. When you go for this hearing test, it is important that you respond as accurately as possible. Do not try to make your hearing loss appear worse than it is.

At some point during this test, you will be asked to repeat a series of single syllable words at a level that is comfortably loud to you in a quiet listening environment. However, you should also request that the audiologist give you this test while you are wearing your hearing aids and listening at a normal conversation level in a noisy listening environment. This type of test will more accurately show the difficulty you will experience when you are listening to a teacher in a college classroom, and will more accurately represent your hearing disability.

You must also have a medical evaluation completed by a doctor that specializes in diseases of the ear to assure that you do not have a medically treatable hearing problem. In addition, you will need a general medical evaluation (unless you have had one in the past year) and a vision test to make certain that you do not have any other medical problems that could interfere with your ability to work. VR will pay for all these tests.

2. Hearing loss as a vocational handicap

Once it is established that you have a hearing loss that is not medically treatable, your VR counselor must determine if your hearing loss is a vocational handicap. In other words your VR counselor must determine if this hearing loss prevents you from getting or keeping a job that you could get or keep if you did not have the hearing loss. While financial status and job market are taken into account, much of this determination is made subjectively by your VR counselor.

3. Potential to benefit from VR services

Before you become eligible for VR services, it must be determined that you can benefit from these services and become successfully employed. Your counselor will look at your previous school performance. It is certainly to your advantage if previous educational history looks good.

Your counselor will evaluate your interests, intellectual abilities, and emotional strengths. Your counselor will be looking at your ability to set realistic goals for yourself. Do not choose a profession where excellent hearing is essential. Choose a profession where you can succeed. Often you will be asked to do a comprehensive job market survey before choosing your career. Suggestions for completing this type of survey are given in Chapter 14.

Your counselor must also determine if you have additional disabilities that could prevent you from becoming employable.

During the formal evaluation process, you will meet several times to discuss your counselor's findings, and explore various vocational goals. Your counselor will discuss the effect your hearing loss might have on the duties of your selected occupation. For example, if you are thinking about becoming a public-school teacher, your counselor might ask how you expect to hear students in the back of the room or how you would react to students that mumble so you cannot hear them. Be prepared to answer such questions. Your answers will help your counselor determine how well suited you are to a particular occupation.

If you feel some of the decisions made by your VR counselor are unfair, discuss your feelings with your counselor. If you still do not feel you have been treated fairly, talk with the VR office supervisor or the Director of the state VR agency. As another alternative, you can discuss your concerns with the state's Client Assistance Program (CAP) office. The address and phone number of your state CAP office can be obtained at the VR office. CAP has been established in each state to negotiate disagreements between VR counselors and VR clients. However, CAP counselors request that you first voice your concerns directly to your VR counselor. Often by simply stating your concerns to your counselor you can resolve the problem. Suggestions for getting what you want from VR counselors and others are given in Chapter 12.

Eligibility

After your counselor determines that you meet the three eligibility requirements, and you have agreed on an occupation that meets your needs and abilities as determined by the formal evaluation, you will receive an Eligibility Certification. The Eligibility Certification shows that you are now a "full-fledged" VR client. At this point you and your counselor are ready to begin writing the Individual Written Rehabilitation Plan (IWRP).

Preparing the IWRP

In this chapter we will only discuss IWRPs for people who are in Status 18. The services that are offered in Status 14 and 16 are usually incorporated into Status 18 for college students who are hearing impaired.

After completion of your formal evaluation, you and your counselor must decide what will be done to achieve your educational and career goals. Financial responsibilities and timetables must be established.

Your counselor will ask you to look for additional sources of financial aid for college to help offset VR expenses. These additional funding sources might include both local and national financial aid programs as well as work-study programs at the college. While you are not required to apply for government loans, you may choose to do so, since the VR agency will have you living on a tight budget. After you have examined a variety of alternate funding sources, you and your counselor will establish in writing the amount of financial support that will be provided by VR. For example, if you plan to attend a state university for four years, VR may pay for your tuition and books, while you agree to pay for room and board. Some students receive money from Supplemental Security Income (SSI) to help pay for room and board. SSI money is provided by the federal Social Security Administration to eligible students who are disabled. If you and your counselor feel that you might be eligible for SSI, contact one of the local Social Security Administration offices in your state for application procedures.

In addition to outlining your financial responsibilities on the IWRP, you must also develop a timetable for reporting your monthly school progress and end-of-semester grades. Generally, to continue VR eligibility you must maintain at least a "C" grade-point average. As stated previously, it is important to show your VR counselor that you are a responsible student. This means that your monthly school reports and semester grade reports should be turned in on time. The timetables and responsibilities are your contract. VR keeps up its portion of the contract by paying for a portion of your college training and providing counseling and job placement services. You must turn in reports on time and get good grades. Doing so will assure your success as a VR client, and will help you develop good habits that facilitate your professional success after graduation.

Job Placement and Post-Employment Services

Your VR counselor can offer a variety of services that will help you find employment in your chosen career. Your VR counselor can help with job hunting, and will help you develop job-interviewing skills. If necessary, your counselor will help develop your résumé. The good news is that most college graduates quickly find a suitable and stable job. After sixty days in this job, your counselor can close your file as rehabilitated in Status 26. Further services can be provided in Status 32 if you encounter difficulties in your new job. To get such services, you will need to contact your VR counselor and make such a request. Your counselor will then reopen your file and determine what is needed to keep you employed. If you move to another state after you graduate from college and then require post-employment services, you will need to contact the VR agency in that state for further services. Either way, VR offers you valuable job placement and job maintenance services.

Conclusion

The state VR agency has a lot to offer college students who are hard-of-hearing. Before you begin college your VR counselor can help you focus on a future career that is right for you. During your college career, VR can help finance your education, and your VR counselor can help you develop job-hunting skills. After college graduation, your VR counselor can help you find a suitable and stable job that will allow you to achieve your full vocational potential. If necessary, further services can be provided after you become employed if you encounter difficulties in your new job. Thus your VR agency has something to offer you throughout your academic and professional life.

The checklist below has been provided to help you get started in the VR process. Hopefully, this information will help you as it has thousands of other college students who are hearing impaired.

Checklist for Obtaining VR Services

_____ 1. Contact the local VR agency in your area to set up an appointment with an RCD or counselor who has previously worked with people who are hearing impaired.

_____ 2. If a group appointment is scheduled for you, request an FM or loop system or a one-to-one meeting.

_____ 3. Develop a list of the technology you need and the professions that are of interest to you. See chapters 4, 5, 8, and 14 for help with this.

_____ 4. If possible, bring any hearing and hearing aid test results that you have received within the past year.

_____ 5. Be on time for all scheduled appointments. Dress professionally, as you would for a job interview.

_____ 6. Provide, in a timely fashion, all information requested by your VR counselor.

_____ 7. If you receive VR funding, keep your grades up.

_____ 8. Inform your VR counselor of any problems you have with your college classes.

References

Architectural and Transportation Barriers Compliance Board (1982). Minimum guidelines and requirements for accessible design. Federal Register, Wednesday, August 4, 33865–33868.

Department of Health, Education and Welfare (1977). Nondiscrimination on the basis of handicap. Federal Register, Wednesday, May 4, 22676–22701.

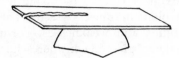

Chapter 8
Getting Ready for College: The Where, When, and How of Succeeding

Grace E. Olmstead, M.Ed.

Preparing to Go to College . . . When and How

The high-school student with hearing loss may have some special needs; however, that fact should not alter the decision-making process of selecting a college or university. The student must examine all of the same issues other students consider (such as location, cost, entrance requirements, etc.), while not overlooking those few extras which are essential due to his or her hearing loss (such as class size, availability of note takers, priority registration, support group, etc.).

College Is Quite Different from High School

In high school, many programs and services are arranged for the student by school officials. Most often, services are even provided in the same building where the student's classes are located. However, once the individual becomes a college student, it is his or her own responsibility to request services, to seek information, and to locate the needed resources.

Another way that college differs from high school is the pace and amount of course work. College courses progress at a much faster pace and demand more reading and writing than do high school classes. The material or information presented over an entire year in high school may be taught in six weeks or less in a college course. College professors work fast, and students must keep up. Students can compensate for the rapid pace and increased work load of college courses by taking less hours (courses) during the term, or by enrolling in subjects which evenly represent the student's academic strengths and weaknesses. Fortunately, the student has some options when planning his/her school schedule.

Another college—high school distinction is that the student is responsible for the purchase of all textbooks and supplies; such a purchase could cost hundreds of dollars each term. In addition, if the student fails a course or wishes to repeat it for a better grade, he/she must pay to take the course again.

The Common Sense of College Selection

Much preparation goes into getting ready for college, and many of the arrangements must be made well in advance of high school graduation. Early in the planning stages, certain aspects of college selection should be given full consideration:

1. The selection of a college should not be based solely on the individual's hearing impairment. Instead, place the emphasis on the student's academic qualifications, desire and motivation to succeed in college and, lastly, the disability.

2. What size school would be most comfortable? Larger schools may provide greater opportunities, but they are more impersonal. Smaller colleges, on the other hand, typically have the advantage of smaller class size.

3. At the midpoint of the junior year in high school, the prospective student and his or her parents should realistically explore what is involved in financing a college education.

How to Afford College

1. Many students may elect to attend colleges in their own communities, in order to keep costs down by living at home.

2. The possibility of obtaining a scholarship should always be explored. A scholarship is financial aid awarded to a student by a college and/or other organization. Many high schools, churches, private groups, businesses, and college financial aid offices have the information necessary to apply. In the case of a college financial aid scholarship application, it is advisable to make a notation indicating "individual with hearing impairment." Many schools have scholarship funds which are designated specifically for students

with disabilities. In fact, some may only be available to individuals with hearing loss.

Researching potential scholarships should begin in November of the student's junior year in high school. Develop a resource sheet including the following data: name of the scholarship, name and address of the contact person, deadline for the application, and eligibility requirements. Gathering this information early will help the prospective student establish a timetable for collecting the required information (e.g., a high school transcript, reference letters, writing a personal essay) and submitting it in time to be considered for a scholarship.

3. The college financial aid office should be contacted early in the student's senior year of high school to obtain information about applying for state and federal grants, school loan programs, etc.

4. It is wise to make an appointment with the local Bureau of Vocational Rehabilitation. This state agency may have a slightly different name depending on the state; however, most telephone directories will list it under state agencies (see Chapter 7). The Bureau of Vocational Rehabilitation (BVR) is a service bureau of the Rehabilitation Services Commission, a state agency responsible for the rehabilitation of those state citizens with physical, mental, or emotional disabilities.

   One of the primary purposes of BVR is to provide to individuals with disabilities the education and/or training that will allow them to be self-sufficient and employable. Once a student is approved for its services, the Bureau of Vocational Rehabilitation may pay a portion or all of the student's college costs, e.g., tuition, housing, transportation, books, hearing aid.

5. If financing is a problem, it is important to keep in mind that state institutions (any public institutions supported and controlled by the state) are usually less expensive than private colleges. However, for out-of-state students, tuition at state schools may also be higher.

Ways to Evaluate Potential College Choices

While keeping in mind the size and cost factors, the prospective student must now begin to establish a list of possible college choices. Try to limit the list to five institutions. It is recommended that the student visit the high-school or community library and study some of the college selection resource books. (See reference list at the end of this chapter).

In addition, the high-school counselor may have helpful materials available.

Once the list of potential colleges has been completed, it is time to study each school in more detail. Use the following as a checklist for evaluating schools, with other criteria added if needed.

I. Entrance Requirements
    A. Is there a specific high-school grade point average required to qualify for admission? The grade point average for entrance will range from colleges with very strict requirements to those with more liberal standards. Some schools have an "open admission" policy. Open admission is a policy for admitting all students regardless of their academic record.
    B. Is there a median SAT or ACT score for entering freshmen? *Median* is an adjective used to describe the midpoint between highest and lowest scores. The American College Tests (ACT) are standardized tests used by many colleges and universities as part of their undergraduate admissions testing program. The Scholastic Aptitude Test (SAT) is a test developed by the Educational Testing Service for the College Entrance Examination Board. ACT and SAT scores are used for college admission decisions and college counseling. Tests are usually taken by twelfth-grade high-school students.
    C. Does the institution specify a certain class rank in its requirements? Class rank is the class standing or relative position of a student in his/her graduating class.
    D. What is the application cutoff date? This is the latest date that an application for admission will be accepted.
    E. Are certain high school courses required for entrance, e.g., foreign language, mathematics, sciences, etc.

II. **Career Goals**
    A. Does the college have academic programs—majors—which correspond to the student's occupational and career goals? A *major* is a term used in an institution of higher education to describe a student's main subject area of specialization.
    B. Does the college have two-year or four-year programs? The two-year program offers two years of college-level work. The student follows an organized curriculum leading to a formal award, such as an associate's degree. The four-year program offers four years of college-level work, culminating in a bachelor's degree. The curriculum may be in either the liberal arts

or sciences, in one or more professional fields, or in both categories.

   C.   Taking a minimal full-time load each term, how long will it take to graduate?

III. The Institution (college or university)

   A.   Consult each institution to determine their full-time status. Full-time status may vary from school to school.

   B.   Is it an accredited school? If the answer to this question is no, remove it from the list immediately. The student needs to BEWARE that not all colleges, trade schools, bible schools, community colleges, business colleges, or institutes are approved by national licensing agencies; nor are all programs within a given college approved. That is, it would be unfortunate to spend time and money on a program, only to find that a job is not available because the profession in question does not recognize that particular training program or school. It would be equally tragic to find that the courses taken at one college will not be accepted for transfer to another. There are many accrediting agencies, so accreditation is an ambiguous issue, yet a crucial one. See your high school guidance counselor or vocational rehabilitation counselor for advice.

   C.   What is the size of the student population?

   D.   What is the cost per term? (tuition, books, supplies, fees, room and board, cost of travel to and from home, etc.)

   E.   Where is the school located—the geographic area?

Investigate the Willingness and Ability of Potential Schools to Provide Services to Students with Hearing Loss

Many individuals with hearing loss have learned to compensate and feel that their hearing loss poses no problems. They are, therefore, convinced that it is not necessary to share information about their hearing loss with outsiders. Please realize that **a college campus is not the place to conceal your hearing impairment.** A pretender might be viewed by instructors and other students as being indifferent, unprepared, withdrawn, unfriendly, or uncooperative, when in fact hearing loss has interfered with the reception of important information. Certainly no person going into a new environment would want to be perceived in this manner. The prospective student should be honest about the disability and not ashamed to communicate his or her needs.

**TABLE 8-1. FORM LETTER EXAMPLE: REQUEST FOR
INFORMATION ABOUT ACCOMMODATIONS**

Blank University
504 Chester Road
Pittsburgh, Pennsylvania 15221
March 1, 1990

Dear Service Provider's Name:

　　My name is Linda Brown and I am interested in attending (Name of School) beginning (School Term and/or Month and Year). The admissions office has provided me with most of the general information regarding your institution.

　　I have a hearing loss and would appreciate any information you can provide regarding services available through your office. Enclosed you will find a list of the accommodations and modifications which would be beneficial to me. Your earliest response and return of this inquiry would be greatly appreciated. I would welcome any suggestions and/or printed materials.

　　Thank you for your time and assistance. If additional information is needed, I can be reached by mail or telephone at 412-376-0736.

Sincerely,
Linda Brown

Each admissions office at the schools under consideration by the student should be contacted regarding the designated department and specific person that provides support services for students with disabilities. The student should remember that the name of the department may differ from institution to institution, e.g., Special Services for the Disabled, Student Services for the Handicapped, Special Student Services, etc. Next, the student could write a form letter and a list specifying needed or desired accommodations. (See Tables 8-1 and 8-2) Such a letter and a list will assist the service provider at the college in determining if the student can be accommodated by the college.

This letter should contain services which have contributed to the success in high school of the individual with hearing loss. This letter might also include other types of assistance which may not have been offered in high school but would have been of value. College is a different ball game than high school. Services may not have been needed in high school, but due to the more impersonal nature of college, larger class sizes, poor classroom acoustics, and the very fast pacing of coursework, support services may be greatly needed in college. Table 8-2 details potential, valuable accommodations for the student with hearing loss.

**TABLE 8-2. A SAMPLE LIST OF ACCOMMODATIONS FOR
STUDENTS WITH HEARING LOSS**

Accommodations/ Modifications	Service Provided by Office	Not Provided by Office	Can Be Arranged	Not Available on Campus
1. Listening/Amplification Systems Provided for Classroom Use and Other Campus Facilities (Auditoriums and Theaters)				
2. Notetakers				
3. Carbonized Notetaking Paper				
4. Permission to Tape Class Notes				
5. Academic Tutoring				
6. Is There a Speech and Hearing Clinic on Campus?				
7. Priority Registration/Assistance with Registration				
8. Telephone Amplifier and/or TTY/TTD for Campus and Dormitory Use?				
9. Do any of the televisions in the dormitories have Closed-Captioning?				
10. Do any of the videotaped instructional materials have Closed-Captioning?				
11. Oral, Cued Speech, or Sign-Language Interpreters				

12. What other services are available for students with hearing loss?

_____

13. Are there any organizations or clubs on campus for students with hearing loss?

_____

The student may want to schedule an appointment with his or her high-school counselor, high school teacher, audiologist, etc., to seek additional recommendations, because these professionals might have a perspective not considered by the student.

Using the information he or she has collected, the prospective student is now ready to develop the form letter and the needs list. The letter should be brief and precise. The disability-related needs list should be put on a separate sheet of paper, so that it can be filled out easily and returned once it has been completed by the service provider.

Before making a final decision about which college to attend, it might be wise for the individual to discuss the selection with his or her parents and high-school counselor. Last but not least, if at all possible, it is always a good idea to visit the college before making the final selection. Do not go unannounced. Call and make appointments to talk with representatives from the Admissions Office, Handicapped Student Services, and Office of the Residence Halls if on-campus housing is being considered.

What Are Your Rights Under Federal Law?

During the last ten years, an increasing number of postsecondary institutions have designated a specific person or persons to provide and manage services for students with disabilities. As a result, college students with disabilities typically receive better and more integrated education services than in the past which enable them to develop their potential more fully.

In September, 1973, the 93rd Congress passed Public Law 93-112, the Rehabilitation Act of 1973. Section 504 of the Act stated: "No otherwise qualified handicapped individual in the United States . . . shall, solely by reason of his handicap, be excluded from the participation in, be denied the benefits of, or be subjected to discrimination under any program or activity receiving Federal financial assistance."

In May 1977, the Department of Health, Education, and Welfare issued regulations implementing Section 504. This nondiscrimination statute and the regulations issued under it guarantee a right of entrance for students with disabilities into our nation's colleges and universities, as well as their participation in the college program as a whole.

The following crucial information, reprinted directly from the *Handicapped Persons Rights Under Federal Law Handbook*, January 1987, U.S. Department of Education, Office for Civil Rights, Washington, D.C. 20202, describes the federal regulations as they apply to colleges and universities.

Section 504 applies to all recipients of federal financial assistance from the Department of Education. Recipients include state education agencies, elementary and secondary school systems, colleges and universities, and state vocational rehabilitation agencies.

The regulation covers only those persons with disabilities who are otherwise qualified to participate in and benefit from the programs or activities receiving federal financial assistance. This coverage extends to persons who are disabled as well as persons who have a history of a disabling condition and persons perceived by others to be disabled.

Postsecondary institutions receiving federal assistance have specific obligations with regard to students with disabilities:

- *Students with disabilities must be afforded an equal opportunity to participate in and benefit from all postsecondary education programs and activities,* including education programs and activities not operated wholly by the recipient.
- *Students with disabilities must be afforded the opportunity to participate in any course,* course of study, or other part of the education program or activity offered by the recipient.
- *All programs and activities must be offered in the most integrated setting appropriate.*
- *Academic requirements must be modified, on a case by case basis, to afford qualified students with disabilities an equal educational opportunity.*
- *A recipient may not impose upon students with disabilities rules that have the effect of limiting their participation in the recipient's education program or activity;* for example, prohibiting tape recorders in classrooms or guide dogs in campus buildings.
- *Students with impaired sensory, manual, or speaking skills must be provided auxiliary aids,* such as taped texts, interpreters, readers, and classroom equipment adapted for persons with manual impairments.
- *Students with disabilities must have an equal opportunity to benefit from comparable, convenient, and accessible recipient housing, at the same cost as it is available to others.*
- *Students with disabilities must have an equal opportunity to benefit from financial assistance.* A recipient may not, on the basis of disability, provide less assistance than is provided to nondisabled persons, limit eligibility for assistance, or otherwise discriminate.
- *Students with disabilities must have an equal opportunity to benefit from programs that provide assistance in making outside employment available to students.*
- *Students with disabilities must be provided an equal opportunity to participate in intercollegiate, club, and intramural athletics.*

- *Students with disabilities must be provided counseling and placement services in a nondiscriminatory manner.*

Special Services for the Disabled

It is the responsibility of the designated office, which may be called Disabled Student Services or Handicapped Student Services, to develop and coordinate support services for the student population with disabilities. As previously discussed, adjustments and accommodations for the student with hearing loss may include, but not be limited to: tutoring; note takers; priority registration; oral, cued speech, or manual interpreting; TTY/TTD; special listening/ amplification devices for classroom lectures; etc. In addition to providing these services, the director or coordinator is usually the liaison between the college and outside service agencies such as the local or state rehabilitation agencies.

When seeking services, there are two very important rules to remember and practice:

1. If the services you require are *not* among those offered, always ask the Director or Coordinator of Disabled Student Services for what you need.
2. Be accepting of your hearing loss—do not try to hide it. If you are uncomfortable with your hearing loss, others will sense the discomfort and may react to it. Be confident and promote yourself.

Colleges and universities offer many services to all of their students free of charge. Some of these may include personal counseling, career planning, health services, speech and hearing services, and on-campus job placement (employment while in school).

Academic Advising

Colleges or universities may differ in their approach and system of providing academic advising. Regardless of the system the institution has adopted, it is important to recognize the value of academic advising. The adviser can provide *accurate* information regarding:

1. **Major Requirements**—each college or university demands the completion of specific courses and/or credit hours in order for a student to qualify for subject specialization;
2. **Course Prerequisites**—a requirement/requirements which must be taken and successfully completed prior to enrolling in a course;

3. **Curriculum**—a term not only including the program of studies, but also all the experiences that a learner has in a school which will help him/her to reach the institution's broad goals and objectives;

4. **Recommended Credit Hour**—A unit used by institutions of higher education to measure/record academic work successfully completed by students. A specific number of credit hours is assigned to each course, this reflecting the number of clock hours spent in class each week and the number of weeks in the academic term. Graduation requirements specify the number of credit hours to be completed for a given academic degree;

5. **Load Per Term**—the number of credit hours or courses a student is registered for during the term.

However, it is important to remember that the adviser is there to provide direction, furnish the facts, and to advise, not to make decisions for the student.

The student should be candid with the adviser about his or her hearing loss. He or she should not be afraid or ashamed to ask questions. Most advisers would rather have a student ask questions so that the adviser may know that the student has a clear understanding of the information. If, after listening to the adviser's response, the matter still is not clear, ask that the information be repeated. Do not walk away without a clear understanding of the facts.

Selecting a Major

First it should be stated that all students do not enter college having decided upon a major. In fact, the opposite is probably true. A high percentage of students entering college for the first time are undecided about a major field of study and remain undecided for several years. Statistics also reveal that the average student changes his or her major at least twice during the college career. So don't feel bad if you don't know what you want to be; most of us don't.

When attempting to make a career choice, it is important to consider the following factors:

1. **Career goals and interests.** The student should first give consideration to a major which is directly or closely related to his or her career goals (see Chapter 14 for more information).

2. **Areas of academic strengths and weaknesses.** The student must be realistic about his/her academic abilities. For example, no in-

dividual should attempt to major in engineering if he or she has a history of weakness in mathematics and science.

3. **Job availability after graduation.** It is essential that the student investigate the future outlook for employment opportunities in his or her area of specialization. Consideration should be given to the geographic location where the student would like to reside and work after completing school. This information can be provided through the academic department, job placement office on campus, and/or the public library.

4. **Possibility of obtaining work experience on campus or in the community in the student's chosen field, prior to graduation.** On-the-job work experience is an excellent way to explore career-related goals before finishing college. Examples of two such college programs are **Cooperative Education**, a formal educational program which combines classroom study with on-the-job experience in a paid, academically-related employment position (all colleges do not have this type of program); and **Internship**, an extended field experience normally carried out under the direction of a training institution and scheduled as the culminating part of a professional training program. The purpose of the internship is to provide the trainee with on-the-job training under the supervision of an experienced practitioner and/or a university supervisor. The student may discover that he or she has the academic aptitude for the field but does not like the working conditions. Such work experience in the student's selected career area will be a valuable asset once the student has graduated and he or she is competing in the job market.

Surviving Registration

The days of standing in long lines to register for classes have become a thing of the past at most institutions of higher learning. With the onset of the era of technology, schools now have the option of employing more expedient systems. For example: mail registration and telephone registration.

Regardless of the method adopted by the college, it is the responsibility of each student to personally register for his or her courses. Because most courses have an enrollment limit, it is important that the student *know and respect* the established *deadlines* and pay attention to registration details.

The student may wish to inquire in the Office of the Registrar as to his or her *designated time to register*. For example, some schools register their students according to their class rank (freshman, sophomore, junior, and senior) while others may use an alphabetical system.

Priority registration, a service which allows students with disabilities to register for their classes early and thus avoid being "closed-out" of needed courses, is available at many institutions. Inquiries about this special service should be directed to the Office of Disabled Student Services.

Once the student with a hearing loss has determined the appropriate registration dates, he or she should *make an appointment with the academic adviser*. Meeting with the adviser should not be a last minute effort, because the student and/or the adviser may need time to seek additional information relating to course selection and/or other significant matters. *Students should not register for courses without first consulting their academic adviser. In addition, the student with hearing impairment should consult the Office for Disabled Services to arrange the needed support services for the coming term.* If the student is receiving any type of financial aid, he or she should also visit that office before completing registration.

As already indicated, schools may differ in their method of registration. Therefore, it is *essential that the student read all registration materials*. All schools provide some type of printed information which usually includes course offerings for the next term, times and location of courses, the registration schedule (beginning and ending dates), and other registration instructions. The student should consult the Office of the Registrar for such printed material.

Summary

Hopefully this chapter, "The Where, When, and How of Succeeding," will assist the student with hearing loss in making the transition from high school to college.

The student should use the college experience as a building block for the future. Remember, aside from the academic knowledge obtained, both positive and negative experiences have value in the learning process that will prepare one for the world of employment after graduation. While in college, students with hearing loss are encouraged to take risks and to investigate new opportunities. In the protective college setting, students will have access to trained personnel to offer guidance when confusion and/or conflict arise.

Summarized below are issues which were discussed in this chapter. These suggestions are meant to aid the student with hearing loss throughout his or her college experience; they are also meant to encourage the student's development and ability to accept responsibility after graduation.

1. Students with hearing loss are encouraged to take the time to find a college or university that can meet their academic and personal needs.

2. Do not hide your hearing loss from instructors and friends.

3. Students planning to go away to school must assess the cost (tuition, room and board, books, and all the extras) and review financial resources with their family.

4. While you are in college it is important to learn to budget your time wisely.

5. The Federal regulations as they apply to universities and colleges are outlined in this chapter, and every student with a hearing loss is encouraged to read them.

6. There are many university support services available to students; use them!

7. All students must learn the value of reading the materials the college provides, e.g., registration information, fee deadlines, course requirements, fees, school disciplinary policies, and the student newspaper. Remember the phrase, "ignorance is no excuse." A hearing loss is no excuse for not knowing the policies and procedures.

References

Jarrow, J., Baker, B., Hartman, R., Harris, R., Lesh, K., Redden, M., & Smithson, J. (1986). *How to Choose a College: Guide for the Student with a Disability*. Washington, DC: HEATH Resource Center.

Lehman, A.E. (1987). *Annual Guide to Undergraduate Study Four-Year Colleges, 1987*. Princeton, NJ: Peterson's Guides.

Lehman, A.E. (1987). *Annual Guide to Undergraduate Study Two-Year Colleges, 1987*. Princeton, NJ: Peterson's Guides.

Liscio, M.A. (1986). *A Guide to Colleges for Learning-Impaired Students*. Orlando, FL: Academic Press.

MacMillan Co. (1985). *The College Blue Book*. New York: MacMillan Co.

Marquis Professional Publications. (1984–5). *Yearbook of Higher Education: A Directory of Colleges and Universities*. New York: Marquis Professional Publications.

Ready Reference Press. (1980). *Directory of Information Resources for the Handicapped*. Santa Monica, CA: The Press.

Straughn, C.T. & Straughn, B.L. (1983). *Lovejoy's College Guide*. New York: Monarch Press.

Thomas, C.H. & Thomas J.L. (1986). *Directory of College Facilities and Services for the Disabled*. Phoenix, AZ: Oryx Press.

U.S. Department of Education. (1987). *Handicapped Persons Rights Under Federal Law Handbook*. Washington, DC: Office for Civil Rights.

Van Cleve, J.V. (1987). *Gallaudet Encyclopedia of Deaf People and Deafness*. New York: McGraw Hill Publishing Co.

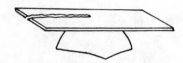

Chapter 9
Studying and Learning: Helpful Services Your College May Provide

Mary King, M.A.

The purpose of this chapter is to explain what the college entrance process is like and to describe what students should look for in the way of academic support services when considering colleges. Basic skills courses, tutoring services, and learning skills labs or centers are commonly provided in colleges concerned about the academic welfare of students. Will only students with hearing impairments resort to these services? Absolutely not! Here's why:

The University Environment

A university is very much a verbal environment. Lectures, class discussions, directions for taking tests, textbooks, and the tests themselves are given to students in words, which students must hear or read. In a way, reading is easier than listening, since most of us are able to read more words than we use in conversation. We are more likely to *recognize* words in print than words that are spoken to us, though recognizing words does not by itself guarantee that we will understand a passage when we read it, if the concepts are new ones. But when we are listening to long sentences that contain new concepts, it's very hard even to *hear* unfamiliar words well enough to identify them. Students are likely to lose the thread of meaning while taking notes. Then, when they ask questions during or after class, the professor may answer in language which is loaded with words unfamiliar to the beginning student (Figure 9-1).

113

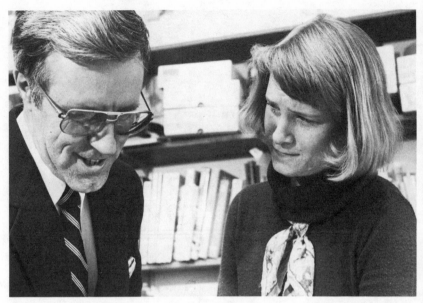

Figure 9-1: Such Words as Syllabus, Thesis, Fallacy, and Analysis are Commonly Used by College Teachers, Who Don't Realize that the BewilderedFreshman Doesn't Know What's Being Said.

The Thicket of Words

The student is caught in a thicket of verbal density, a mass of words packed with meanings vitally important for him or her to understand in order to act on them. Also, the student has never heard these words before, and therefore can't even remember them to look them up later or ask someone what they might mean, much less do whatever he or she is being told. The student may nod and smile, hoping for a dignified escape from the conversation, but still needing information.

The impact of this verbal density is so great that many students with normal hearing make verbal errors that are silly, embarrassing, and costly. Here is what happened to one freshman working on an assignment for his English composition class. Darryl came into the Writing Lab with a paper based on an interview he had conducted with a professional in his field, accounting. He explained that he'd learned a lot from the interview, that being an accountant was much harder and more complicated than he'd realized. He read several pages of his draft aloud, with no mention of accounting. Finally, he identified his interview subject as a "sales accountant executive," and it became clear that he had heard the word *account* as *accountant* when his subject gave him her job title. Fortunately, desk dictionaries define *account executive*, so he could see what term she had actually used. This student error is not really surprising, though he would have been embarrassed if he had not realized his mistake in time to correct it.

Cognitive Overload

Such mistakes are often caused by cognitive overload, a situation where the mind is occupied with too many concerns at too many levels and can't attend to them all simultaneously. On one level, Darryl was thinking about his assignment, which was complicated in itself, as we'll see in a minute. But at the same time, because he was new to the University, he was preoccupied with adjusting to a new life. He was still learning his way around the campus. He hadn't figured out when to do his laundry. He felt loaded down carrying too many big textbooks around all day, but he wasn't sure which ones he needed for class, so he brought them all. He missed his old friends and felt uncertain about making new ones.

With all these concerns (and who knows what others?) Darryl simply didn't listen closely to his interview subject at a crucial moment, the moment when she told him her job title. He heard the word that fit into his needs and expectations (accountant) because his overriding need was to produce a paper that would satisfy the assignment. Finding an accountant was only the first step. He then had to arrange an interview while recording it in writing or on tape, select from his recorded material that which was relevant to the assignment, and write the paper, making it as correct as possible.

The fact that this student with normal hearing had this problem understanding what was said to him shows that the language environment at college challenges the abilities of many students. In fact, everyone has problems understanding the words of new areas of learning, and for people with hearing impairments the problems can be especially damaging, actually threatening your ability to succeed. You'll find more discussion of problems with hearing in Chapter 2. At any rate, because students flounder a bit at first, most institutions of higher education provide a more or less complete academic support system.

Starting Out Behind

In view of the abstractness and density of language used in universities, and in view of the student's need to master these academic language habits, it would appear that "starting out behind" is the rule rather than the exception for entering college freshmen. Indeed, according to a survey of all colleges and universities in this country, conducted by the City University of New York,

> A full 85 percent of the 1,269 responding institutions perceive poor academic preparation of incoming freshmen to be either very much of a problem or somewhat of a problem.
> A substantial percentage of entering freshmen are viewed as requiring assistance in the basic skill areas—28 percent in reading, 31 percent in basic writing, and 32 percent in basic mathematics (Lederman, Ryzewic, Ribaudo, 1983, p.1).

But remember, these statistics are just another way of saying that students have a lot to learn. So we shouldn't feel discouraged—*of course* students have a lot to learn. That's why they're in school. And that brings us back to the subject of this chapter: How does the institution determine that a particular student is not well prepared academically? And what kinds of support do schools provide to help these students learn what they need to learn?

Placement Testing

First off, most schools test their incoming freshmen in the traditional skills: reading, writing, and arithmetic. Such testing is done during an orientation day, before students sign up for classes. This way, the tests can be scored before students meet with their advisers, so the advisers know what courses are appropriate for individual students.

Reading

Almost all schools that test reading use multiple-choice tests, which include sections on comprehension of brief passages and on vocabulary. The reading passages may range in length from single paragraphs to several pages of factual material on different subjects. For example, one such test includes two paragraphs of music history followed by five questions. Two of the questions ask the reader to remember details—or find them, since the reader is permitted to look back at the passage. Three questions ask the reader's understanding of the passage as a whole: What is the main idea of the second paragraph? For which purpose was the first paragraph written? Which principle underlies both paragraphs?

Answer sheets are provided; these may be scored by machine. Since these are timed tests which ask only that you choose among answers that have been provided for you, they obviously cannot reveal all there is to know about your reading. But tens of thousands of college students have taken these tests, so your score can place you quite accurately within broad categories. Your reading score may influence the decision about your English placement and may also indicate that you should take a course in college reading and study skills.

Writing

Most schools assess writing by means of a writing sample. This means that students meet in a room where paper, pencils, and space for writing are provided. A topic is presented to them, and they are given a specified amount of time, usually half an hour to an hour, in which to write on that topic. Commonly, these placement writing tasks require the writer to relate a personal experience and to explain why and how it was significant. In most schools, two trained teachers rate the whole set of papers in a single session. Occasionally both a writing sample and a test of grammatical or mechanical correctness are given. A few schools test only for correctness, in a multiple-choice, true-false, or fill-in-the-blank format, but this is *not* an adequate test of writing.

Scores from these writing samples help the academic advisers place students in one of three groups: those who should take honors English or go directly into an advanced course; those who will be able to learn what they need to know about college writing in the standard English composition course; and those who need instruction and practice in writing before enrolling in English composition. This last group will take Basic Writing as their first writing course in most colleges. As you can see, these are fairly broad categories, so placing students within them is not a difficult matter.

Mathematics

Testing in mathematics usually covers the general skills of addition, subtraction, multiplication, and division as well as basic algebra. Many schools create their own tests; some use a test package produced by Educational Testing Service.

Unlike the reading and writing tests, the math test is one you can prepare for by reviewing and practicing what you have studied in school, especially such basic skills as working with fractions, decimals, and percentages. If you don't refresh your knowledge, you may score low on the test just because of a rusty performance. Your low score will look the same as the score of someone with less advanced study in math, and you'll be placed the same.

Since accurate placement is very helpful for students, you should view the testing process as a useful one—the best way for you to get to the courses where you can succeed. You should not be surprised if you score in the lower categories in reading and writing; hearing impairments make it difficult to learn and use language well. But neither should you be discouraged. A good school for you will provide courses and tutoring to help you catch up. Remember, too, that the test scores are not the only information your adviser will have. Your high school grades and SAT or ACT score will contribute to the overall picture, and of course, you will be able to talk about your educational experiences with your adviser.

Basic Skills Courses

Good **basic skills courses** are as different from poor ones as talented drummers are from beat machines, so ask what these courses are about and how they are taught as you investigate the college you are considering. Overall, here are some features to look for: small classes, peer collaboration, concentration on the skills area, and minimal testing.

• **Class size** is important because large groups tend to isolate individuals and permit them to avoid coming to grips with the problem at hand—as you know from high school experiences. The social relationships that can be fostered in smaller groups encourage purposeful learning. Fifteen or twenty students are plenty in basic skills courses.

• Peer collaboration is an unfamiliar term for a very fruitful approach to learning that is discouraged in high schools—namely, working with your classmates instead of competing against them. Collaboration means cooperation—helping one another other understand the material and produce your best work. It places responsibility on the learner—you.

• It sounds silly to say that **basic skills** classes should concentrate on the skill area—but not everyone agrees on what's *basic* in basic skills. Many so-called basic writing courses are really courses in grammar, spelling, and punctuation, even though experts in the field agree that people learn to write by writing. A course that requires lots of guided writing practice will teach you more about writing than a course in which you spend most of the time studing parts of speech. Likewise, in a college reading course, you should be doing plenty of reading and responding to what you read in class discussion and in writing. The same goes for math, obvious as it sounds. These courses have to be *intensive*—

meaning *you* have to practice the subject, using the skill yourself, to learn how to do it.

• Therefore, too much testing is to be avoided because testing takes time from actually doing your reading, writing, and arithmetic. Frequent quizzes, especially in math, are probably useful to keep you alert to your own progress; and in reading, too, other kinds of performance opportunities should be provided than too-frequent all-period, knock-down, drag-out tests.

In spite of all the work basic skills courses require, at many schools you cannot earn college credit for them; they are regarded as preparatory courses. Be prepared for this possibility and find out in advance, so you can't be disappointed. Whether or not you can earn college credit by taking basic skills courses, plan on working as hard as you would for a credit course—or even harder! You may find, for example, that you will do more writing in your Basic Writing class than in English Composition.

Learning Skills Centers or Labs

Many students are surprised to learn that to be successful in college, they must spend one or two hours on coursework outside of class for every hour they spend in class. This means that a "normal" fifteen-credit load actually takes up fifteen to thirty hours' study time in addition to fifteen hours in class. In other words, thirty to forty-five hours' time must be spent on school work each week. So a full-time student is working at school work as much as a full-time worker works at a job. And this is the case for *all* students, not just for those with special problems.

Learning skills centers or laboratories (labs) can be very helpful here, showing you how to spend your time fruitfully. (The term *lab* and *center* mean the same, but some schools use one and some use the other.) If you were fortunate enough to attend a high school that provided a writing center, you will come to college already knowing how and when to seek out the writing consultants who can work with you as you practice writing. Most colleges have writing centers, and they are becoming more common in high schools. Centers or labs for math and for reading and study skills are less frequent, but look for them in the colleges you consider, and plan to utilize them on a regular basis.

What a Basic Skills Center Provides

The professional staff of a basic skills center can meet with students by appointment to discuss, on an individual basis, the difficulties you are having with your coursework. These are teachers, graduate students, or trained peer tutors familiar with your courses and with the level of performance that is expected of you. But they are not your classroom teachers, and they don't judge or grade your work. Rather, they can go behind the product of your work—the test answer or essay—to the **process** you used to produce it, and help you find ways to improve the product. Such analysis is very different from the kind of instruction that goes on in most classrooms and can get at the sources of your problems more easily than is possible in classroom settings.

In writing, for example, your teacher can't tell why your five-hundred-word theme is only a page long, doesn't fulfill the assignment, and is full of errors but empty of information. And you may not feel like explaining that you hadn't the faintest idea what the topic meant when it was assigned or what you should do to respond to it, so you put it in the back of your mind for five days, worrying about it but not writing; then at midnight just before the paper was due, you tried to write it up, but each attempt was more off the wall than the last, so at 3:00 a.m. you decided to abandon the project and hand in what you had. Your teacher may suspect that's what happened, but will almost certainly be too polite to say so; after all, there are so many other possible explanations of how this paper came to be. Donald Murray, a highly respected teacher of college writing, identifies the classroom teacher's difficulty, and it's all too true: The person reading a piece cannot imagine what actually went on in the writing process. Learning skills centers exist to get behind that sausage and take a look at what happened to the pig.

Writing Centers

In a writing center you can talk about and practice figuring out how to approach assignments. You can practice the kind of writing expected of you with a skilled consultant available to teach you at points where you need information. And you can ask the writing center tutor to use an Assistive Listening Device (ALD; see Chapter 5) so that you can more easily hear how your paper sounds when you read it aloud, and you can use your own language skills to help you with writing. Your own speech and your tutor's speech are more intelligible with the use of the ALD because both of you are speaking directly into the unit's microphone. With the ALD you can also hear more clearly what your tutor says about your writing. The combination of individual attention to your writing and an enhanced ability to hear can be very helpful to you in improving the clarity and correctness of your writing.

Reading/Study Skills Centers

Similarly, in a reading/study skills center, you can present the problems you're having with textbooks to a skilled reading specialist who will help you direct your attention more efficiently as you study and take tests. Many of your teachers will give you good advice about using your textbooks well and studying effectively, but often because of the pressure of comprehending the material of the course, students can't attend to such advice. Having opportunities for guided practice outside of the classroom can be very helpful.

Math Centers

In math, too, the student and teacher are disadvantaged in the classroom. The class must move forward, whereas individual students may need to be taken backwards to find out the reasons why misunderstandings occur and to clear up confusion and errors in reasoning. Such matters can easily be managed in the more leisurely, open setting of a math center.

Peer Tutoring

An excellent service offered by many colleges is peer tutoring in specific courses. Peer tutors are students who have succeeded academically, so in addition to helping you learn the subject they're tutoring, they can teach you quite a bit about being a good student. They also know how to get things done, like applying for financial aid, using the campus health services, and finding material in the library.

Find out early how to apply for a tutor, and put in your application early in the semester. If you wait too long, you may find there are no more individual tutors available.

Peer tutors, basic skills center staff, teachers in your basic courses—all will show you what to practice and how to practice. Hard work is something American students aren't very good at, compared to students in other countries, but we can learn. The National Academy of Sciences released a study in January, 1987, comparing American grade and secondary school achievements in mathematics with those of students in other countries. U.S. students ranked among the lowest of any industrialized country. In identifying reasons for U.S. underachievement, researchers mentioned a powerful difference in attitudes about what produces academic success.

"The Japanese and Chinese believe that people are basically the same and that the difference between success and failure lies in how hard you work," according to Harold W. Stevenson, professor of psychology at the University of Michigan. "Americans give more importance to native ability, so they have less incentive to work hard in school" (Fiske, 1987, p. 10).

Success for students with hearing impairments comes from having that attitude that makes them put a lot of effort into their schooling and take responsibility for their own learning. With the support of basic skills courses, basic skills learning centers, and peer tutoring, students with hearing impairments can find considerable success in college. Many of them do well, by dint of sheer hard work. In fact, as a person with a disability, you may have an edge on "normal" students, who sometimes don't know what hard work is. At any rate, don't let your hearing impairment be an excuse for poor achievement. It needn't be.

Checklist of Academic Support Services

The college or university that is concerned about the welfare of its students will provide services to help all its students learn how to work hard in school. Services which are vitally important to those with hearing loss include the following:

- **Placement testing** tells your adviser what courses you need to take.
- Basic skills courses give guided practice in reading, writing and arithmetic.
  Small classes allow lots of feedback on your work.
  Collaborative learning means you work with your fellow students, developing confidence and a sense of responsibility.
  Ample practice of the target skill promotes your growing competence.
  Minimal testing tells you your strengths and weaknesses without taking too much time away from the work of the course.
- **Basic skills learning centers** provide professional teachers or peer tutors to work individually on your difficulties with reading, writing, or math.
- **Peer tutoring** provides skilled fellow students to help with problems in particular courses.

Remember too, to **use an Assistive Listening Device (ALD)** in each of these settings (see Chapters 5 and 6 for details). An ALD is easy to use and essential for increasing your learning.

Use these services—you won't be alone. Rather, you'll find yourself in a whole learning environment, immersed in the teaching-learning process with other highly-motivated students aiming for success.

References

Fiske, E. B. (1987, January 11). U.S. Pupils Lag in Math Ability, Three Studies Find. *The New York Times*, pp. 1, 10.

Hawkins, T. (1976). *Group Inquiry Techniques for Teaching Writing*. Urbana, IL: National Council of Teachers of English.

Lederman, M. J., Ryzewic, S. R., Ribaudo, M. (1983). *Assessment and Improvement of the Academic Skills of Entering Freshmen Students: A National Survey*. (Research Monograph Series Report No. 5) New York: Instructional Resource Center, Office of Academic Affairs, City University of New York.

Additional Reading

Ender, S. C., McCaggrey, S. S., Miller, T. K. (1979). *Students Helping Students: A Training Manual for Peer Helpers on the College Campus*. Athens, GA: Student Development Associates.

Foster, E. S. (1983). *Tutoring: Learning by Helping*. Minneapolis: Educational Media Corporation.

Margeneau, J., Sentlowitz, M. (1977). *How to Study Mathematics*. Reston, VA: National Council of Teachers of Mathematics.

Olson, G. A. (Ed.). (1984). *Writing Centers: Theory and Administration*. Urbana, IL: National Council of Teachers of English.

Schaier, B. T. (Ed.). (n.d.) Critical issues in tutoring. New York: NETWORKS, Bronx Community College.

Shollar, B. (1982). *Tutoring Reading and Academic Survival Skills*. New York: Longman.

White, E. M. (1985). *Teaching and Assessing Writing*. San Francisco: Jossey-Bass.

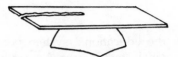

Chapter 10

The Role of the Speech-Language Pathologist: They Don't Still Need Speech Therapy, Do They?

Denise Wray, Ph.D.

In view of the fact that a speech-language pathologist is one of the major members of the professional team in higher education that provides assistance for students with hearing loss, such students must realize what the speech-language pathologist can do for them. The pathologist is not there simply to assist with speech-sound improvement. This professional's role is gradually expanding to include many areas not traditionally serviced by the speech-language pathologist. The remainder of this chapter will outline and describe the services that fall under the responsibility of this professional. These responsibilities include, but are not limited to, serving as:

- Advocate for the college student with a hearing impairment
- Liaison with the Office of Handicapped Student Services and other university faculty
- Cosupervisor and creator of a support group
- Referral source for other needed services
- Speech-sound therapist
- Language therapist (including teaching basic writing skills)
- Educator of basic hearing aid and hearing equipment care

Advocate for the College Student with a Hearing Impairment

Most students venturing through the educational system occasionally need a person to speak on their behalf, to advocate. Generally, this individual is a parent until students are sufficiently skilled and confident to begin taking over these responsibilities themselves. A student with hearing loss encounters many more dilemmas than hearing peers during the school years. For instance, the use of current amplification technology may have required inservicing to teachers and peers by speech-language pathologists, audiologists, or parents. Taunting from other students is often an issue and may have to be dealt with by a parent or teacher. Parents are usually accustomed to regular contact with school personnel and oftentimes parents play this role all too well and run the risk of becoming overly protective. Further, if the parent does not assume this responsibility, who will? It is hoped that parents recognize the importance of gradually shifting some of the duties onto the students themselves. Developing the confidence to effectively approach a teacher or educate a friend will build invaluable skills for later life. In fact, some students feel very comfortable in voicing needs and requests to teachers, peers, and administrators. As many will admit, advocating is well worth the effort.

Unfortunately, much of that assertiveness goes by the wayside once students with hearing loss enter a higher-education environment. Unlike the elementary-and-secondary-school years, parents cannot be used as "back-up troops" to forge the way into the more difficult situations. On the contrary, parents may be the individuals least familiar with the domain of higher education. Things may have changed drastically since they went to school. Furthermore, one may wonder, what assistance, if any, is available for the student with hearing loss?

The fact of the matter is, not only is assistance available, but "accommodations," as federal law refers to them, are mandated for any institution receiving federal funding (Jenkins, 1981). Granted, the laws are interpreted and put into action in ways which differ from one university or college to the next; however, they do exist. The students' task is to locate an institution which is willing to best serve their particular needs (see Chapter 8). Once in that setting, it is advisable to seek a new advocate immediately; someone who can facilitate independence. This should be someone who knows the specifics of the law at the higher educational level, and who has a sincere commitment to the attainment of educational goals by students with hearing impairments. This role may best be served by a speech-language pathologist or audiologist on the faculty in a department of communicative disorders.

The student with hearing loss should contact the Department of Communicative Disorders immediately and locate the individual faculty member who coordinates services for students with hearing impairments. If a coordinator does not exist, this may be an indication that there is a weak link between the Department of Communicative Disorders and the Office of Handicapped Student Services.

The speech-language pathologist and/or audiologist may also be able to explain how the Department of Communicative Disorders can assist a college student with hearing loss. Services typically offered by this department include:

- Audiological assessments (hearing tests)
- Hearing aid evaluations and troubleshooting
- Speech-language services
- Information on state-of-the-art assistive technology
- Equipment loans (varies greatly from institution to institution)

Liaison with the Office of Handicapped Student Services and with Faculty

In a related vein, some requests may best be handled by the Director of Handicapped Student Services (see Chapter 8). All federally funded institutions must have someone who oversees students who experience disabilities. As mentioned earlier, if the Department of Communicative Disorders and the Office of Handicapped Student Services work together or appear to communicate with one another, this is a very favorable sign. This interdepartmental communication becomes especially evident when difficulties arise with the instructor of a student who is hearing impaired. When classroom difficulties occur, correspondence may extend beyond the Departments of Communicative Disorders and Handicapped Student Services. It may be necessary to contact a professor of a student who is hearing impaired to clarify assignments or to review errors made on previous examinations. At The University of Akron, if extended test time, interpreters, notetakers, or tutors are requested by a student, he/she must first approach the Director of Handicapped Student Services. If clarification of lecture notes or test questions is required, or other areas are queried that the Director feels are under the realm of speech-language or audiology, the student is immediately referred to the Department of Communicative Disorders. Students are referred to the audiology faculty member for technical matters, such as hearing aid problems, ear-mold fittings, updated amplification, hearing assessments, hearing aid evaluations, etc. These responsibilities are very time consuming. Thus, the speech-language pathologist takes on more of an advising and coordinating role that may often entail frequent referrals to the audiologist.

Cosupervisor and Creator of a Support Group

The benefits of support groups have been touted in the literature (Berg, 1972). There is nothing so therapeutic as sharing and empathizing with others who have experienced similar trials and tribulations in life. This is particularly true for those students with hearing loss who have led largely a mainstreamed life. Many of these students reported that they had very limited contact with peers with hearing impairments (Flexer, Wray, & Black, 1986). Thus, Drs. Flexer and Wray created a support-information group in Spring, 1983, for college students with hearing loss attending The University of Akron. The group continues to meet twice a month and participation is voluntary (see Chapter 13). The reader may wish to refer to Chapter 15 which is authored by college students with hearing loss themselves. Note the frequent reference to the therapeutic function of the support group. The message is clear: SUPPORT GROUPS *DO* MAKE COLLEGE LIFE EASIER.

It is suggested that the audiologist and speech-language pathologist cosupervise the group because of the nature of the target goals. For example, training in troubleshooting, updating of audiograms and amplification, earmold difficulties, etc. (see Chapter 2), make it mandatory that sufficient audiologists be available to fulfill requests of students with hearing loss. Once the students recognize the value of the support group, they will use the services frequently, and both the audiologist and speech-language pathologist are "on call." Perhaps the best promoters of a support group are the students themselves. One out-of-state student with hearing loss attending The University of Akron explained the impact of the group on his life:

> "After coming to these meetings for several years, I am
> not ashamed of my hearing loss. And best of all, it's not a
> "taboo" subject in my family. I always felt like family mem-
> bers were speaking in hushed voices behind my back, afraid
> of embarrassing me. In fact, that's just what they did by never
> mentioning the hearing loss in my presence."

Referral Source for Other Services

Although the speech-language pathologist and audiologist may attempt to be all things for all students with hearing loss, there are times when student needs fall outside the purview of these professionals. An example of an opportune time to refer to another professional is the case of students who may be going through an emotionally turbulent time in their lives. Students with hearing loss may be withdrawn or isolated from peers (Davis, Elfenbien, Schum, & Bentler, 1986) and placement in a hearing college setting may only intensify those behaviors. Guide them away from questionable groups that solicit lonely students on campuses. Rather, refer them to a reputable counselor, psychologist, or psychiatrist. Oftentimes, free counseling services are available on campuses that have training programs in this area. If professional counseling is not a viable alternative, another option is a referral to another student with hearing loss who may have experienced similar difficulties earlier. Sharing with someone who has "been there before" can mean a new beginning for a student feeling like a "misfit" in the fast paced and complex university environment.

Lastly, it goes without saying that the most important referral the speech-language pathologist may make is to the audiologist. Indeed, the speech-language pathologist is responsible for simple acoustic and visual inspections of hearing aids and other equipment. However, whenever there exists an iota of doubt, call in the audiologist! Students with hearing impairments cannot afford to be without proper amplification. Undue auditory disadvantages should not be imposed on students who already have enough pressure in the classroom.

Speech-Sound Therapist

This chapter differentiates goals that may be speech-sound related from those that are language-based. Speech-sound goals work on correcting the production of sounds that one may say in error such as "r" or "s." Language goals, on the other hand, deal with difficulties the student with hearing loss may have with understanding the vocabulary or complex sentence structure of the English language.

Improving speech-sound production may be a low priority for a student with hearing loss. After years of therapy, many are reluctant to have "more" therapy. However, following adoption of new amplification or the latest in earmold modifications, a student who could not previously hear a high frequency sound may be able to do just that for the first time. Incorporation of this new sound into conversational speech may occur rapidly or may require intense lessons of drill, practice, and auditory monitoring. If a student is interested in continuing to improve speech, he/she should be enrolled in therapy. As long as the motivational force exists, the prognosis is generally good.

Who should deliver the service—the speech-language pathologist? The audiologist? Aural rehabilitation may be provided by the speech-language pathologist with the consultation of an audiologist. It depends on the working assignments arranged by these two professionals. Some audiologists may not feel comfortable delivering services of this type, or they may simply not have the time (Wilson-Vlotman & Blair, 1986). Generally, one professional is designated at the "expert" in this area and schedules the clients accordingly.

Assessment of Speech Sounds

Prior to explaining evaluation and speech sound intervention procedures, the author would like to include several comments. First, this book's philosophical orientation toward habilitation for individuals with hearing loss is very aural in nature; accessing hearing is the first strategy employed (Ling, 1989). That is to say, the student's hearing is maximized through state-of-the-art amplification fittings followed by the student being taught to use his/her residual or remaining hearing to the greatest extent. To determine the existing phonetic skills of the student and those which should be targeted for therapy, one of the first tests administered is the *Phonetic Level Speech Evaluation* by Daniel Ling (1976). This tool assesses suprasegmental aspects of speech, vowels and dipthongs, single consonants at four various levels and consonant blends in both initial and final positions. A thorough evaluative tool, it provides numerous phonemes that could potentially be targeted for therapy. The speech inventory by Ling will at least indicate what the student can do and under what conditions (i.e., given various phonetic combinations and environments), and it provides an excellent starting point for therapy.

Intervention

Daniel Ling's (1989) phonetic level speech training outlines a carefully sequenced program for the speech-language pathologist or audiologist. A sound is selected for pairing with another sound based upon its acoustic structure and on its ability to enhance correct production of the target.

Emphasizing the auditory characteristics of target sounds that lie within the student's amplified hearing range may be a novel experience for many speech-language pathologists or audiologists. They may be accustomed to resorting to "watch me" cues when the target sound is in error. The clinician may wish to highlight audition through use of a personal FM System during therapy. An FM with a good high frequency response can more easily emphasize these characteristics, particularly for voiceless fricatives such as "s", "f," and "sh," due to the use of the remote microphone (see Chapter 5). These and other therapy concepts are best illustrated in one of Ling's videotapes on speech training or any of his published books.

Language Therapist

The negative impact of hearing loss on learning to understand and use language is documented sufficiently in the literature to alert the speech-language pathologist and audiologist (Brackett & Maxon, 1986; Davis, et al., 1986; Ross, Brackett, & Maxon, 1982). Even a mild hearing loss can adversely affect academic performance (Blair, Peterson & Viehwig, 1985). Hearing serves as the foundation for acquiring language skills such as speaking, reading, and writing (Ling, 1989). Acknowledging the research that places the person with hearing loss at high risk for language disorders, professionals cannot assume that language difficulties are "outgrown" by college. The college environment requires high level, refined language skills such as oral recitation, debating, verbal explanation, and demonstration of a variety of written literary types.

Receptive Skills

Comprehension of colloquial and formal textbook terminology encountered in college may be far below age level. One must never assume the student with hearing loss understands all the vocabulary presented in conversations, directions, or in reading material. Commercial programs that target vocabulary concepts are acceptable to use, but preferably only as a supplement to the student's own textbooks and other reading materials. If goals are not practical and useful to the student's course of study, the purpose of language therapy becomes "fuzzy" to the student and motivation in therapy quickly wanes.

Writing Skills

Writing literacy is an essential skill for successful academic achievement, particularly at the level of higher education (Kelly & Whitehead,

1983; Suhor, 1984). Students with hearing impairment are in danger of developing disorders in terms of language acquisition (Davis, 1977; Davis & Hardick, 1981; Ross, Brackett, & Maxon, 1982) due to what is called the "acoustic filter" phenomena (Ling, 1989). Simply put, hearing is the basis of verbal language development. Progressively, deficits in the area of oral language could negatively affect the higher level language skills of reading, writing, and ultimately academic achievement (Simon, 1985; Wallach & Butler, 1984).

At The University of Akron, speech-language pathologists and audiologists use a team approach to meet the language needs of college students with hearing impairment (Flexer, Wray, & Black, 1986). Initially, these students sought services to improve speech-sound production, but standardized testing revealed significant language deficits, particularly in the area of writing. The fact is, there is little in print that can guide the speech-language pathologist or audiologist when establishing a program for writing intervention. A more in depth description may be found in *Language, Speech & Hearing Services in the Schools* (Wray, Hazlett, & Flexer, 1988).

On the surface, writing may appear to be a visual task; however, it is dependent on one's verbal language and reading skills (Holbrook, 1984). Developing a solid basis for spoken language and a good intrinsic feel for its rule system sets the stage for adequate competence in writing.

The strategies employed by the speech-language pathologists and audiologists at The University of Akron Speech and Hearing Center, are a combination of theories derived from research completed on normal hearing students and those with hearing impairment.

Previous attempts at teaching writing to students had focused little on the techniques good writers actually use to write. That is, students had never been taught how to begin a paper, draft, focus on the audience, set goals, revise, and edit. Rather, they were given a particular literary type (e.g., descriptive paper, compare/contrast, expository) and simply told to reproduce a similar one. Not knowing how to arrive at the end product and having their attempts red inked, resulted in students viewing writing as an exercise in teacher-imposed torture.

Fortunately, the research produced by such authors as Donald Murray (1982), Donald Graves (1979, 1983), and Lucille Calkins (1982) has begun to change the philosophy of compositional writing and ultimately the attitudes of student writers. Their approach is one that is known as the "process" approach that stresses the fact that writers go through numerous stages before arriving at a suitable end product. Much regard is given toward planning, re-thinking, and focusing on ideas, goals, and the audience. While grammar is attended to later in the process, it no longer is the central theme as in a traditional approach to writing.

Five major stages of the writing process will be discussed with the highlights of each stage briefly outlined below.

Auditory Considerations Stage

In view of the importance of maximizing hearing in an auditorily stressed program, certain factors must be considered before directly teaching writing skills. First, achieving the best auditory input, particularly for high pitch sounds like "s" and "sh," was a primary objective, providing that the student had high frequency residual hearing. This often required a referral to the audiologist for modifications to the student's hearing aids and earmolds in order to better amplify the high pitch sounds. Another way the audibility of sounds was determined was by means of the Ling 5-Sound Test (Ling, 1989). If the student could not easily detect all 5 sounds, an FM auditory training unit was employed in an attempt to emphasize all sounds. Thus, maximizing the student's hearing often entails frequent technical advice from a skilled audiologist.

Pre-Writing Stage

The beginning steps in creating a written piece of work involve pre-writing activities. These can include anything from drawing, observing, reading, brainstorming, to "doodling," mapping, or interviewing (Tompkins & Friend, 1985). The writer simply puts pen to paper to generate a variety of ideas. At this point no attention is given to grammatical conventions, spelling, and other mechanic-related items.

Drafting Stage

Once the information is written down, it is time to organize the material in a more cohesive manner. Therefore, the student begins to focus on the main topic and supporting sub-topics of the paper. Keeping this in mind, the manuscript is either expanded or reduced in certain areas. One technique which aids in organizing the major topic from its supporting points is mapping. Mapping visually outlines the major thrust of the paper and easily illustrates which ideas legitimately support the main topic and which are irrelevant (see Figure 10-1).

It is during the drafting stage that students are required to read their papers orally numerous times in order to develop a "sense" of how the paper sounds in terms of content. Peer conferencing also takes place at this time with a friend or clinician listening to the oral readings followed by routine questions such as, "What are you trying to say in

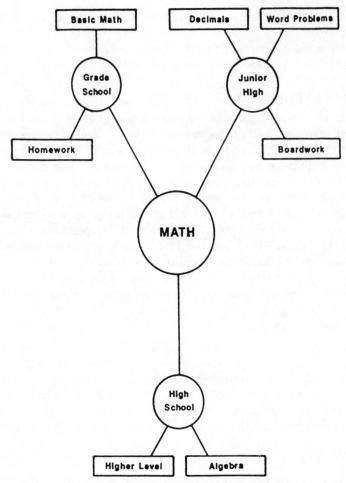

Figure 10-1: Mapping Technique Depicting Major Theme of a Paper with Supporting Subtopics.

this paper?'' or ''How does that paragraph relate to the purpose of the paper?''

Revising/Editing Stage

Once the content of the paper begins to shape up, the mechanical aspects that one usually associates with writing begin to be addressed in addition to continual improvements in content. If, following the oral readings, students are still unable to identify errors in verb tense, pluralization, word usage, etc., the clinician may use certain cues. For instance, the clinician may mark the margin of the paper to indicate the general vicinity of an error. Or, questions can be posed which offer the student some guidance in pinpointing existing errors.

Final Drafting Stage

This is often referred to as the "clean-up" stage because it involves extensive attention to punctuation and grammar. Now is the time for the student to dwell less on content (for the first time in this process) and more specifically on the visual components that make up a paper such as punctuation, spelling, and mechanics.

Grammatical checklists which pinpoint problem areas specific to the student are introduced. Grammar areas that are repeatedly violated are included on the checklist such as commas, verb tense, verb endings, possessive markings, etc.

Finally, reference books such as the dictionary, thesaurus, and a speller are employed extensively during this stage. Thus, it is imperative that the student with hearing loss be skilled and well-versed in the use of these resources.

In summary, receptive skill instruction and strategies in writing development are the primary goals targeted for college students with hearing impairment. Language therapy can serve to enhance the students' opportunity to succeed during the beginning years when they are still learning coping skills.

Education in Basic Hearing Aid and Hearing Equipment Care

After reading Chapters 3, 4, and 5 dealing with technological strides achieved in the area of hearing impairment, the benefits of hearing aids and assistive listening devices are obvious. While the audiologist is the expert in technological management, the speech-language pathologist needs some basic skills in order to perform highly effective therapy (Woodford, 1987). The speech-language pathologist's dedication to the belief that appropriate and optimal amplification is critical in a student's aural rehabilitation program presents its own set of challenges. Unfortunately, the inoperable state of hearing aids in the classroom has been repeatedly reported in the literature (Bendet, 1980). Consequently, the necessity for the speech-language pathologist to learn the basics in hearing aid monitoring and maintenance is underscored. This section will discuss the most basic of maintenance information for amplification systems used by one of the team members, the speech-language pathologist.

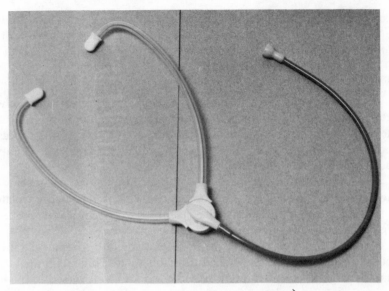

Figure 10-2: Hearing Aid Stethoscope with Rubber Tip Adapter.

Equipment for the Speech-Language Pathologist

Day-to-day monitoring of hearing aids and related equipment is a responsibility that generally is not assumed by any one professional. Only 10 percent of educational audiologists perceived themselves as the individuals who should primarily monitor hearing aids in the classroom (Wilson-Vlotman & Blair, 1986). Ideally, the students themselves will begin to assume the responsibility of their hearing aid care. Certainly, the speech-language pathologist also must be able to demonstrate simple auditory and visual inspections of hearing aids to the students.

In order to conduct basic auditory and visual inspections, several pieces of equipment are a "must" for the speech-language pathologist. The first is a **hearing aid stethoscope** with a rubber tip adaptor that fits easily over an earmold (see Figure 10-2).

This is essential for conducting a good auditory inspection of the hearing aid. A simple listening check should also include repetition of the Ling 5-Sound Test to determine fidelity of the speech sounds: "u,a,e,sh,s". One should pay particular attention to the clarity of the high frequency "sh" and "s" sounds and any unusual extraneous noise being generated. If these appear the least bit suspicious, turn the aid over to an audiologist for an electroacoustic analysis and more thorough inspection.

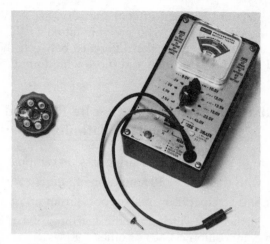

Figure 10-3: Hearing Aid Batteries and Battery Tester.

The second recommended piece of equipment is a **battery tester** that can indicate if a hearing aid battery is weak or dead (see Figure 10-3). Ross, Brackett, & Maxon (1982) cited batteries as a most frequent source of inoperable hearing aids. Surprisingly, some college students cannot recognize a dead battery in their aid (Flexer, Wray, & Black, 1986). The third piece of equipment that may be used on occasion by the speech-language pathologist is a **pipe cleaner** for the cleaning of earmolds or tubing on behind-the-ear hearing aids. Thorough cleaning, if necessary, should *only* be conducted by an audiologist. However, keeping pipe cleaners on hand could prove to be a simple remedy for clogged ear wax in earmolds or tubing.

In the event that the speech-language pathologist has any doubts, he/she should consult an audiologist. This professional specializes in hearing aids and hearing aid equipment care. If listening devices are used in the classroom, it might be added that most of these FM systems come equipped with a helpful troubleshooting manual.

Thus, the appropriate operation of all amplification systems used by the college student with hearing loss cannot be overemphasized.

Summary

The purpose of this chapter has been to illustrate the diversity of services that can be provided by the speech-language pathologist. The point to remember is that a Department of Communicative Disorders devoted to meeting the needs of college students who are hard-of-hearing will have faculty who can offer many services. Audiologists and speech-language pathologists who are committed to the person with hearing impairment can mean the difference between those students who succeed in higher education and those who do not.

Checklist of Services That Can Be Provided by the Speech-Language Pathologist

1. Advocate of students with hearing loss on campus.
2. Liaison with the Office of Handicapped Student Services.
3. Creator and cosupervisor of a support group on campus.
4. Language therapist, including the teaching of writing skills for English composition classes or other courses.
5. Referral source for audiological assessments, hearing aid assessments, and other needs best served by other professionals.
6. Teacher of basic hearing aid care.
7. Team worker with the audiologist.

References

Bendet, R. (1980). A public school hearing aid maintenance program. *The Volta Review, 82,* 149–155.

Berg, F.S. (1972). A model for a facilitative program for hearing impaired college students. *The Volta Review, 74,* 370–375.

Blair, J., Peterson, M., & Viehweg, S. (1985). The effects of mild sensorineural hearing loss on academic performance of young school-age children. *The Volta Review, 87,* 87–93.

Brackett, D., & Maxon, A. (1986). Service delivery alternatives for the mainstreamed hearing impaired child. *Language, Speech, and Hearing Services in Schools, 17,* 115–125.

Calkins, L.M. (1982). When children want to punctuate: Basic skills belong in context. In R.D. Walshe (Ed.), *Graves in Australia* (pp. 89–96). Exeter, NH: Heinemann Educational Books, Inc.

Davis, J. (Ed.) (1977). *Our forgotten children: Hard-of-Hearing Pupils in the Schools.* Minneapolis, MN: National Support Systems Project and Division of Personnel Preparation, Bureau of Education for the Handicapped, Department of Health, Education, and Welfare.

Davis, J.M., & Hardick, E.J. (1981). *Rehabilitative Audiology for Children and Adults.* New York: John Wiley & Sons.

Davis, J.M., Elfenbein, J., Schum, R., & Bentler, R.A. (1986). Effects of mild and moderate hearing impairments on language, educational, and psychosocial behavior of children. *Journal of Speech and Hearing Disorders, 51,* 53–61.

Flexer, C., Wray, D., & Black, T. (1986). Support group for moderately hearing impaired college students: An expanding awareness. *The Volta Review, 88,* (4), 223–229.

Graves, D. (1979). What children show us about revision. *Language Arts, 56,* 312–319.

Graves, D. (1983). *Writing: Teachers and Children at Work.* Portsmouth, NH: Heinemann.

Holbrook, H.T. (1984). Qualities of effective writing programs. *Eric Digest.* Urbana, IL: Eric Clearinghouse on Reading and Communication Skills.

Jenkins, W. (1981). History and legislation of the rehabilitation movement. In R. Parker & C. Hansen (Eds.), *Rehabilitation Counseling* (pp. 6–12). Boston: Allyn & Bacon, Inc.

Kelly, J., and Whitehead, R. (1983). Integrated spoken and written English instruction for the hearing impaired student. *Journal of Speech and Hearing Disorders, 48,* (4), 415–422.

Ling, D. (1989). *Foundations of Spoken Language for Hearing-Impaired Children.* Washington, DC: The Alexander Graham Bell Association for the Deaf, Inc.

Ling, D. (1976). *Phonetic Level Speech Evaluation.* Washington, DC: The Alexander Graham Bell Association for the Deaf, Inc.

Murray, D.M., (1982). *Learning by teaching.* Montclair, NJ: Boynton/Cook.

Ross, M., Brackett, D., & Maxon, A. (1982). *Hard-of-Hearing Children in Regular Schools.* Englewood Cliffs, NJ: Prentice-Hall.

Simon, C.S. (1985). *Communication Skills and Classroom Success.* San Diego: College Hill Press.

Suhor, C. (1984). Thinking skills in English and across the curriculum. *Eric Digest.* Urbana, IL: Eric Clearinghouse on Reading and Communication Skills.

Tompkins, G.E., & Friend, M. (1985). On your mark, get set, write. *Teaching Exceptional Children. 18,* (2), 82–89.

Wallach, G.P. & Butler, K.G., (Eds.) (1984). *Language Learning Disabilities in School Age Children.* Baltimore, MD: Williams & Williams.

Wilson-Vlotman, A.L., & Blair, J.C. (1986). A survey of audiologists working full-time in school systems. *ASHA, 28,* 33–38.

Woodford, C.M. (1987). Speech-language pathologists' knowledge and skills regarding hearing aids. *Language, Speech, and Hearing Services in Schools, 18,* (4), 312–322.

Wray, D., Hazlett, J., & Flexer, C. (1988). Strategies for teaching writing skills to hearing impaired students. *Language, Speech, and Hearing Services in Schools, 19,* 182–190.

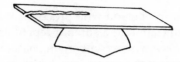

Chapter 11
The Oral Interpreter: The Newest Support Specialist

Winifred H. Northcott, Ph.D.

Current findings show that the degree of hearing loss in an individual of school age does *not* dictate the educational or personal setting in which he or she will be motivated to be competitive, productive, and "turned on" to active learning. (Atkins, 1987; Luterman, 1986; Schildroth & Karchmer, 1986). Today, environments are being created in regular colleges and universities where students with severe and profound hearing losses are performing in proportion to past achievement, innate abilities, and motivation to learn (McCartney, 1987; Saur, Popp-Stone, & Hurley-Lawrence, 1987). Oral interpreting can be part of this new environment.

What Is an Oral Interpreter?

A professionally prepared oral interpreter is a facilitator or an enabler of spoken communication between a person who is hearing and an individual who is deaf or hard-of-hearing, in situations which make it difficult for normal speechreading (lipreading) to take place. Some precise situations come to mind: round-table discussions where rapid shifts in speakers are frustrating, loudspeaker announcements, telephone conversations, voice-only media presentations, facial characteristics of a speaker which obscure clear lip movements, distracting backgrounds, and significant distance between original speaker and the speechreader who is hearing impaired.

What Does an Oral Interpreter Do?

An oral interpreter is usually a hearing person who proceeds at a normal rate of speed and with clear enunciation in a smooth repetition of a speaker's remarks, with or without voice. The accompanying natural gestures and body language help to convey the mood, emotions, and information involved. In a situation where the speech of the individual who is hearing impaired is difficult to understand, the oral interpreter can facilitate full understanding by using voice to repeat what is being said for the benefit of listeners at hand (Castle, 1984; Dirst, 1980; Gonzalez, 1984; Guidelines, 1979; Northcott, 1977; 1979; 1984). The incidental or substantive rewording of a speaker's remarks, while still remaining faithful to the precise meaning of the speaker's words, is the hallmark of the professional oral interpreter.

What Is an Oral Transliterator?

The single distinction between the oral interpreter and the oral transliterator is that the oral transliterator gives a verbatim presentation of the original speaker's remarks, (with or without voice, as the situation requires) whereas the oral interpreter may reword and summarize. The consumer typically indicates his or her preference for transliteration or interpretation during pre-event discussion. Oral interpreters and transliterators do not use sign language during their interpreting performance. Rather, natural gestures, of the sort that one hearing individual would use with another hearing person, and meta-communication are a spontaneous part of oral interpreting or transliterating.

Gonzalez (1988) suggests referring to the oral interpreter or speaker with the feminine pronoun, and the person who is hearing impaired with the male pronoun. The general term "interpreting" is used whether the facilitator presents substantial rephrasing or summarization of the message, or a verbatim rendering of the message.

Hmm, Would an Oral Interpreter Ever be Useful to Me?

The answer to the rhetorical question above is, in part, "know thyself." How well do you hear with or without a hearing aid? Can you position yourself front-and-center of a speaker and gain information directly? Perhaps with the assistance of an FM, infrared, or loop amplification system you have gained even more confidence (see Chapter 5). Only if your hearing aid(s) is malfunctioning and no assistive listening device is available, or the ambient noise level is very high, might you seek an oral interpreter for a particular event.

On the other hand, Eleanor Devine reminds us eloquently that there are others, like herself, "Even with a mic, amplifier, earphones and two hearing aids, I mostly hear mishmash." It all comes down to a consideration of "different strokes for different folks."

The Code of Ethics: An Umbrella of Protection

The presence of an oral or sign language interpreter injects a third party into situations or conversations between a student with hearing loss and his freedom to converse without monitoring. The Registry of Interpreters for the Deaf, Inc. (RID) recognized this from its first year of formal activity, in 1964. At first, the Code was a series of guidelines to govern ethical and professional behavior for the interpreter, the consumer who is hearing impaired, and the hearing person. Currently, the Code of Ethics is a set of standards which describe three basic tenets: confidentiality, impartiality, and integrity. Specifically, the Code states that any interpreter/transliterator shall:

1. Keep all assignment-related information strictly confidential,
2. Render the message faithfully, always conveying the content and spirit of the speaker, using language most readily understood by the person served,
3. Not counsel, advise, or interject personal opinions,
4. Accept assignments using discretion with regard to skill,
5. Request compensation for services in a professional and judicial manner,
6. Strive for further knowledge and skills by participating in workshops and professional meetings, by interacting with professional colleagues, and by reading current literature in the field,
7. Strive to maintain high professional standards in compliance with the Code of Ethics.

Rebecca Carlson, former Director of the Interpreter Training Program at St. Paul TVI, Minnesota, has expanded on the principles of the Code in an eloquent set of illustrations which give some structure and substance to the canons of behavior outlined in the Code (Carlson, 1984).

Help in Locating a Qualified Oral Interpreter

The process of securing a certified oral interpreter will vary from state to state (Castle, 1986; Northcott, 1984). An open-ended list of potential sources for help would include:

- Alexander Graham Bell Association for the Deaf, Inc.
  3417 Volta Place, NW, Washington, DC 20007
  Telephone: 202-337-5220 and TTD
- The Registry of Interpreters for the Deaf, Inc.
  8719 Colesville Road, Suite 310, Silver Spring, MD 20910
  Telephone: 301-608-0050
- state chapters, AG Bell
- state Departments of Vocational Rehabilitation
- state chapters of SHHH, Inc. (Self Help for Hard-of-Hearing People
- a college or university offering workshops in oral interpreting
- a speech and hearing center
- a program or agency serving the hearing impaired
- another speechreader who uses an oral interpreter

Summary

If you are a student with hearing loss, it is important to evaluate your assets, values, and priorities as they relate to the usefulness and/or availability of the newest support specialist; a qualified oral interpreter/transliterator. If you are an interested professional, you have an opportunity to assess the strength of your advocacy role in helping to bring dreams of students with hearing loss into fruition. Remember, the student enrolled in your college or university has EARNED the right to be there. Will you use your credibility and authority to assist him or her in becoming truly assimilated in the academic and social life on campus?

References

Atkins, D.V. (Ed.) (1987). Families and their hearing impaired children. Monograph. *The Volta Review, 89*, (5).

Carlson, R.H. (1984). The Code of Ethics: Some interpretations (221–229). In W.H. Northcott (Ed.), *Oral interpreting: Principles and Practices*. Washington, DC: Alexander Graham Bell Association for the Deaf, Inc.

Castle, D.L. (1984). Effective oral interpreting: An analysis (169–187). In W.H. Northcott (Ed.), *Oral interpreting: Principles and Practices*. Washington, DC: Alexander Graham Bell Association for the Deaf, Inc.

Castle, D.L. (Ed.) (1986). *Oral interpreting: Facts for Consumers*. Brochure, 12 p. Washington, DC: Alexander Graham Bell Association for the Deaf, Inc.

Dirst, R.D. (Ed.) (1980). Oral Interpreter Evaluation Manual for Evaluators. RID National Evaluation System. Silver Spring, MD: Registry of Interpreters for the Deaf.

Gonzalez, K.A. (1984). The content of practicum observation and supervised interaction (pp. 187–221). In W.H. Northcott (Ed.), *Oral Interpreting: Principles and Practices*. Washington, DC: Alexander Graham Bell Association for the Deaf, Inc.

Gonzalez, K.A. (1988). Some thoughts on oral interpreting at the elementary, junior high and high school levels (pp. 15–18). In D.L. Castle (Ed.), *Oral Interpreting: Selections from Papers by Kristen Gonzalez*. Washington, DC: Alexander Graham Bell Association for the Deaf, Inc.

. . . *Guidelines for the preparation or oral interpreters: Support specialists for hearing impaired individuals*. (1979). *The Volta Review, 81*, 135–145.

Luterman, D.M. (Ed.) (1986). *Deafness in Perspective*. San Diego: College Hill Press.

McCartney, B.F. (1986). Factors contributing to the lives of the hearing impaired: Perspective of oral deaf adults. *The Volta Review, 89*, 325–335.

Northcott, W.H. (1977). The oral interpreter: A necessary support specialist for the hearing impaired. *The Volta Review, 79*, 136–144.

Northcott, W.H. (1979). Introduction. In Guidelines for the preparation of oral interpreters: Support specialists for hearing impaired individuals. *The Volta Review, 81*, 135–145.

Northcott, W.H. (1984). *Oral interpreting: Principles and Practices*. Washington, DC: Alexander Graham Bell Association for the Deaf, Inc.

Saur, R., Popp-Stone, M.J. & Hurley-Lawrence, E. (1987). The classroom participation of mainstreamed hearing impaired college students. *The Volta Review, 89*, 263–277.

Schildroth, A.N., and Karchmer, M.A. (Eds.) (1986). *Deaf Children in America*. San Diego: College Hill Press.

PART III-COUNSELING

We all know that the "college experience" involves far more than the acquisition of knowledge. College is a time of emotional growth, a time for developing independence and a new sense of worth. For students who are hearing impaired, college is also a time of coming to terms, once again, with hearing loss.

Chapter 12 is a common-sense discussion of sensitive emotional issues and coping strategies. Chapter 13 tells how to start an information-support group, and why and how this group can facilitate emotional growth. How to plan for a career and life after college is presented in Chapter 14. Finally, Chapter 15 represents the pinnacle of this book with poignant essays written by students with hearing loss who are currently competing in hearing universities. There is no doubt that their hard-won successes deserve a standing ovation.

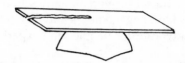

Chapter 12
Coping with Hearing Loss

Ron J. Leavitt, M.S.

The purpose of this chapter is to identify and discuss some of the behaviors that have helped college students who are hard-of-hearing achieve success in their personal and academic lives. If you feel that these behaviors might help you, then you have the difficult job of learning to apply them consistently in your life.

It is easier to discuss the behaviors necessary for success than it is to use them all the time. Learning and consistently applying behaviors necessary for success require practice in a lot of different situations (Trychin, 1987). Do not become discouraged if you decide you want to use some of the behaviors discussed in this chapter and then find that you are not applying them in every important situation. In fact, when you first start using these new behaviors you will often forget to use them in the most important situations because when you are under pressure, newly learned behaviors are forgotten and old behavior patterns are used. Be patient. Consistently using effective coping behaviors in your scholastic and social interactions takes time. The behaviors and ideas described in this chapter are those used by the most successful students with hearing loss I have known. Let me give you an example:

In 1985, I met an eighteen-year-old college freshman named Kim who was very hard-of-hearing. She had never discussed her hearing loss even with close friends or family members. Her earmolds were worn out, and she could not understand a person's speech through her hearing aids unless she was sitting in a quiet room, directly in front of that person. Generally speaking, Kim did not have the tools that are necessary for success in college. Fortunately, Kim believed she could succeed. She started learning about hearing aids and the other technology described in Chapter 5. She started learning about vocational rehabilitation services, disabled student services, and the coping strategies described in this chapter. Today, Kim is a leader in the hard-of-hearing community. She is an excellent student who is involved in many school activities. She has numerous public speaking engagements and has developed a state-wide reputation as an advocate for people who experience hearing loss.

Some might say that the potential for success was within Kim all the time. However, Kim feels that the resources described in this book made her success much easier. Look at the technology and services described in earlier chapters and apply the suggestions for coping with hearing loss offered here. Many college students have benefited from this information. I think you will too. Now, let us look at these suggestions for coping with your hearing loss.

Suggestion 1: Join a Support Group for People Who Are Hard-of-Hearing.

The support group can provide an opportunity for people with hearing loss to learn about available technology and resources (Flexer, Wray & Black, 1986). The group also provides powerful organizational backing for students who are hard-of-hearing to serve as advocates for the technology and services promised to them by federal laws.

In addition to the educational and self-advocacy opportunities offered by the support group, group members can provide emotional support to one another. For example, many students with hearing loss in a support group find it comforting to meet others in the college who share similar problems related to hearing loss. While family members, friends, audiologists, teachers, and counselors with normal hearing can offer a variety of valuable services, only the members of the support group can provide a dimension of understanding and insight not available to people who have normal hearing.

Other emotionally beneficial factors that occur for support group members have been identified by Yalom (1975) and include the following:

1. Learning that occurs while listening to the life experiences of others,
2. Learning that occurs from the advice provided by the group leader and other group members,
3. Development of a sense of belonging or "fitting in" with the group,
4. Development of insight into the causes of a person's emotional "hang ups," and

5. Development of a sense of optimism about future professional and personal interactions.

Ideally, these support group opportunities can be offered on the college campus so they are accessible to all students with hearing loss.

It should be noted that an appropriately trained group leader is necessary so that group experiences are of maximum benefit to all members (Trychin, 1987; Yalom, 1975). Fortunately, group-leader training seminars are currently being offered throughout the country to psychologists and counselors who work with people who are hard-of-hearing. Information about these seminars can be obtained at the following address:

Dr. Samuel Trychin
Department of Psychology
Gallaudet University
Kendall Green N.E.
Washington, D.C. 20002

Support group activities may expand into neighboring communities and result in improved services to people with hearing loss throughout the state. Thus, the development of a support group for students who are hard-of-hearing may bring benefits that extend beyond the campus boundaries.

Suggestion 2: Practice Positive Thinking and Positive Actions.

It has been said that it is aerodynamically impossible for the bumblebee to fly. However, since the bee does not know this, he flies anyway. This aerodynamic miracle attests to the power of positive thinking. Numerous students with hearing loss have become personally and academically successful in college because they believed they could succeed, and their consequent actions brought them success. A student with hearing loss who practices positive thinking and positive actions expects to communicate in every situation. Such a student will request access to all of the college's academic and extra curricular activities as promised by federal regulations (Department of Health, Education & Welfare, 1977; Architectural and Transportation Barriers Compliance Board, 1982; Telecommunications for the Disabled Act, 1984). The students with hearing loss who use positive thinking will use FM, loop, infrared, and audio-input systems as described in Chapters 5 and 6. Such positive thinking and positive actions are crucial to the student's success.

By contrast, negative thinking will result in actions that create failure both personally and academically. Negative thinking causes students who are hard-of-hearing to believe that college officials will not provide essential technology, or that people will not try to communicate effectively with them. Fortunately, such negative beliefs are usually inaccurate. So promise yourself that you will succeed and let your actions guide you to success.

Suggestion 3: Learn to React to Situations in a Way That Helps to Achieve Desired Goals.

Every day you react to thousands of events in your environment. Some of these events are important. Some are not. Often, you feel stress or tension when reacting to the important events. The way you handle this stress often determines your personal, academic, and professional success. If you react in a way that achieves your goals and creates a favorable impression with others, you are successful. If you react in a way that does not achieve your goals, or if you upset others while achieving your goals, you will not be successful. You must learn to react in a way that allows everyone to come out ahead. This can be very difficult. Often when you really want or need something, you forget to think about how you are affecting others. You might become angry if your friends do not speak slowly and clearly in a noisy restaurant. You might feel hurt if your date seems insensitive to your communication needs. These are perfectly normal feelings. However, if you react to these stressful situations by yelling at people or by hurting others, you have not achieved your desired goals.

It is important to remember that people are not "making" you angry or hurting your feelings. You make yourself angry. You allow yourself to feel hurt. People may say or do insensitive things. However this does not automatically make you angry or hurt. Even if you do become angry or feel hurt, you can still choose to react in a way that achieves your desired goals. It is certain that you are more likely to achieve these goals if you treat others with respect and kindness. Do not allow yourself to blow up at people, even if you have to remind them to speak clearly several times. Being a student with hearing loss takes self-discipline. It is not easy. However, when you learn to react to stress in a way that achieves your desired goals without hurting others, you will be more successful.

Suggestion 4: Do Not Allow Unfinished Business to Pile Up.

Perls (1959, 1979) has suggested that unresolved conflicts, unresolved emotional issues, and unfinished work greatly reduce a person's ability to deal effectively with the present. For this reason, Trychin (1987) has recommended that the most "painful" issues for a person be dealt with first in the support group. Whether or not these issues are related to the individual's hearing loss is not a concern. Thus, in both personal and group situations, it is essential to deal with important conflicts, emotional issues, and projects as soon as possible. Otherwise this unfinished business will interfere with every part of your life, including your success in college.

Unfortunately, some people get in the habit of avoiding problems rather than solving them. For example, a person who is hard-of-hearing may learn to dominate conversations rather than trying to understand what other people are saying. Although this behavior may avoid the communication problem, it does not solve it. Communication must be a two-way process. Refusing to follow this unwritten rule will ultimately create serious interpersonal problems.

Another way people allow unfinished business to pile up is to discuss their problems without looking for solutions. While it is important to discuss personal problems with others, it is even more valuable to solve them. In the support group, some members reject good advice from the group. They do not follow logical suggestions and they may introduce other unrelated problems each time a good suggestion is made. The reasons for such behavior are varied and are discussed elsewhere (Berne, 1973; Perls, 1979; Steiner, 1974). However, you should remember that as a successful student with hearing loss, you must learn to develop problem solving rather than problem avoiding strategies (Trychin, 1987). This means dealing with the important events in your life, right now, in a way that will achieve your personal and academic goals.

Suggestion 5: Learn About the Technology Available to People with Hearing Loss. Determine Which Technology Will Help You, and Use it Consistently.

Usually students who are hard-of-hearing benefit from wearing two hearing aids with audio-input and high-fidelity telecoils (Ross, 1977, 1986), and using a notetaker. A frequency modulation (FM) or loop system is also essential. Additionally, a portable telephone amplifier or telecommunication device for the deaf (TDD) and a telecaption decoder are necessary. For personal safety, some type of visual or tactile signal alerting device, as described in Chapter 5, is also desirable (Leavitt, 1987; Leavitt & Freeburg, 1985).

The student with hearing loss who has this technology available has the basic resources necessary to communicate effectively in all educational and personal situations. However, to achieve the best possible communication, the student must use these devices at all times. This can be very difficult and in some instances embarrassing. However, it can be done with the help of a supportive student group (Leavitt, 1985). Without use of the technology described above, the student with hearing loss will spend a considerable amount of time guessing what was said in school and at social activities and will often lose interest in many of the activities that most people find enjoyable. Such loss of mutual interests creates needless isolation for students who are hard-of-hearing. For these reasons, the technology described in Chapters 4, 5, and 6 is considered essential.

Suggestion 6: Learn About Your Legal Rights as a Student with Hearing Loss and Learn How to Obtain What the Law Promises You.

Federal regulations require that FM or loop systems, hearing aid compatible telephones, telecommunication devices for the deaf (TDDs), telecaption decoders, and visual signal alerting devices are to be provided free of charge to students with hearing loss attending public colleges and universities (Department of Health, Education & Welfare, 1977; Architectural and Transportation Barriers Compliance Board, 1982; Telecommunications for the Disabled Act, 1984). However, experience has shown that these devices usually have to be requested by students or they will not be provided. Ideally, these devices will be requested by the entire support group. If the group makes such requests, essential technology is more likely to be provided (Leavitt, 1987).

To further improve the chance of getting essential technology at the college, students with hearing loss should request equipment that they have already tested. One easy way for a group of students who are hard-of-hearing to experiment with a variety of technology is to arrange for a field trip to a technology demonstration center. At these centers, students can experiment with devices that improve speech understanding, telephone communication, and television enjoyment. In this way, the entire student group can determine which technology is most useful. Brochures and pricing information can be obtained at the center. This information can then be used to prepare written proposals for college administrators, describing necessary equipment and projected costs.

Typically, providing college administrators with written requests for essential technology has been sufficient to get this equipment purchased by the college. However, in some rare instances it has been necessary to file a compliance violation against the college with the Regional Office for Civil Rights. Compliance violations may be filed against any public college or university that does not provide FM or loop systems, TDDs, amplified telephones, and signal alerting devices to students with hearing loss.

It should be recognized, however, that filing a compliance violation against the college may create bad feelings between college administrators and students with hearing loss. Such bad feelings make it more difficult for students to achieve future goals. Thus, the filing of a compliance violation should be viewed as an action of last resort. It is preferable to work with college teachers and administrators whenever possible in a way that allows both college personnel and students with hearing loss to benefit from these interactions. In other words, students with hearing loss should assume that college administrators want to provide the technology that is listed above. More often than not, this assumption is true once administrators learn what technology is required by students who are hard-of-hearing.

Obviously, it will take time to become familiar with legal issues and technology available to people who experience hearing loss. It also takes time to meet with administrators to explain requests for technology. However, if you do not become familiar with this information and learn to advocate for yourself, you will always be dependent on someone else to provide you with what you need to succeed in college and in your chosen career. Experience has repeatedly shown that such dependency is not in your best interest.

Suggestion 7: Learn the Rules That Improve Your Ability to Communicate and then Learn How to Get People to Follow Them.

Hodgson (1987), and Matkin and Heald (1987) have developed the following list of rules for improving communication with people who are hard-of-hearing:

1. Get the person's attention before beginning to speak.
2. Face a person with hearing loss directly before beginning to speak.

3. Speak in a normal but strong voice.

4. Enunciate clearly without elaborately mouthing words.

5. Do not eat, smoke, or chew when talking.

6. State the topic to be discussed when starting a conversation.

7. Rephrase sentences that a person with hearing loss has difficulty understanding. Do not repeat the sentence over and over using the same exact words.

8. Speak at a moderate rate of speed with occasional pauses.

9. Check comprehension before changing topics.

10. Use body language and natural gestures.

11. Eliminate unnecessary noise sources such as television or radio when communicating.

12. Do not attempt to communicate from another room.

13. Stand or sit so that the light coming into the room is on your face, not in the eyes of the person who is hearing impaired.

After you have learned these rules you must teach people to follow them. This can be difficult and frustrating. Even after you have taught these rules to teachers, family members, employers, coworkers and friends, they will forget from time to time. This is especially true when people are under stress. Remember that you, too, sometimes forget newly learned behaviors when you are under stress. So be forgiving but persistent. As discussed previously, you should react to others in a way that will help you to achieve your goals. Be careful not to alienate people by reacting negatively when they forget these communication rules.

Videotaped examples of how to teach people to follow these communication rules have been developed at Gallaudet University (see address given previously for ordering this information). This instructional videotape demonstrates "right and wrong" responses to various communication situations and allows people who are hard-of-hearing to practice these behaviors in a number of different situations. Such videotape practice can be beneficial to students, and can be part of the support group activities.

Suggestion 8: Learn to Relax While Listening.

Trychin (1987) reported that 52 percent of adults with hearing loss felt anxious when they were communicating with others, compared to 8 percent of a similarly matched group of adults with normal hearing. Further, college students who are hard-of-hearing often report that they are exhausted at the end of the day after straining to hear their instructors. This is especially true when students do not make consistent use of essential technology (Leavitt & Freeburg, 1987).

To help reduce the tension that students who are hard-of-hearing experience when listening, application of suggestions 5, 6, and 7 is recommended. Additionally, students must learn to relax when communicating.

Suggestion 9: Enjoy Your College Career.

Most successful students spend four to ten years in college. These years will be much more enjoyable if you learn to approach projects with a positive outlook. At college the opportunities for enjoyable educational adventures are everywhere. If you expect to enjoy these adventures, you will. If you expect to enjoy coping with your hearing loss and improving the way you react to others, you will.

Students who are hard-of-hearing often report that their college years are the most enjoyable. Part of this enjoyment has come from learning about themselves, their hearing aids, their legal rights, and available technology. The have also enjoyed developing effective coping strategies as discussed above.

Kenny Rogers said in his song *The Gambler*, "If you're going to play the game, you better learn to play it right." The same thing can be said about going to college. If you are going to spend so many years of your life in college, you should learn to enjoy the time spent. You can, "If you learn to play it right."

Acknowledgements

The author would like to acknowledge the academic contributions of Dr. Sam Trychin and Mr. David Curry. The inspirational contributions of Laura Adams, Betty Bounds-Wood, Jack Cassell, George Kosovich, Kimberly Lindas, Margie Magee-Mori, John McElhinney, Dodie McSorley, Sandy Mintz, Lisa Moshofsky, Bill Mosier, David Viers, and Kim Wood are also acknowledged.

Coping Behavior Checklist

_____ **1.** Join a support group for people who are hard-of-hearing.
_____ **2.** Practice positive thinking and positive actions.

_____ **3.** React to situations in a way that helps to achieve personal goals.

_____ **4.** Do not allow unfinished business to pile up.

_____ **5.** Learn about the technology you need, and use it consistently.

_____ **6.** Learn about your legal rights.

_____ **7.** Learn about the rules that improve your ability to communicate, and help people to follow them.

_____ **8.** Learn to relax while listening.

_____ **9.** Enjoy your college career.

References

Architectural and Transportation Barriers Compliance Board. (1982). Minimum Guidelines and Requirements for Accessible Design. Federal Register, Wednesday, August 4, 33865–33868.

Berne, E. (1973). *Transactional Analysis Psychotherapy: A Systematic and Social Psychiatry*. New York: Ballantine Books.

Department of Health, Education and Welfare. (1977). Nondiscrimination on the Basis of Handicap. Federal Register, Wednesday, May, 4, 22676–22701.

Flexer, C., Wray, D.F., & Black, T.S. (1986). Support group for moderately hearing impaired college students: An expanding awareness. The *Volta Review*, *88*, 223–229.

Hodgson, W.R. (1987). Personal Communication.

Leavitt, R.J. (1985). Counseling to encourage use of SNR enhancing systems. *Hearing Instruments*, *36*, 8–9.

Leavitt, R.J. (1987). Promoting the use of rehabilitation technology. *ASHA*, *29*, 28–31.

Leavitt, R.J. & Freeburg, J.J. (1987). Survey of ALDs interest. *Hearing Instruments*, *38*, 29.

Matkin, N.D. & Heald, M. (1987). Personal communication.

Perls, F.S. (1959). *Gestalt Therapy Verbatim*. New York: Bantam Books.

Perls, F.S. (1979). *Gestalt Therapy: Excitement and Growth in the Human Personality*. New York: Bantam Books.

Ross, M. (1977). Binaural vs. monaural hearing aid amplification for hearing impaired individuals. In Bess, F. (Ed.). *Childhood Deafness: Detection, Assessment and Management*, Chapter 19. New York: Grune & Stratton.

Ross, M. (1986). Classroom amplification. In Hodgson, W. (Ed.). *Hearing-aid Assessment and Use in Audiologic Habilitation: Third Edition*, Chapter 11. Baltimore: Williams & Wilkins.

Steiner, C. (1974). *Scripts People Live*. New York: Grove Press.

Telecommunications for the Disabled Act. (1984). Federal Register, Wednesday, January 11, 1356–1357.

Trychin, S. (1987). Principles of Effective Interaction: A videotape demonstrating four principles of behavior as related to hearing impairment.

Yalom, I.D. (1975). *The Theory and Practice of Group Psychotherapy*. New York: Basic Books, Inc.

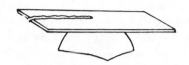

Chapter 13
We're All in This Together: The Support Group for College Students with Hearing Loss

Carol Flexer, Ph.D., Denise F. Wray, Ph.D, Thomas S. Black, M.S.

As noted in previous chapters, special academic and advising services are provided by many universities for students with hearing loss. In addition, audiologic and speech/language services are often available. Nevertheless, it became clear that students were not using, or were unaware of, existing accommodations. Something was missing. There was no unifying force, no efficient way of informing students about resources. Students were telling us that they felt isolated, that they did not know other students who were hearing impaired. The formation of a self-help group seemed to be a logical solution. There were community self-help groups (SHHH) available, but the students felt that their unique and specific needs could not be addressed by a group whose members were older and already in the work force. Therefore, we decided to form our own self-help group as a vehicle for providing emotional support and new information to college students with hearing loss.

How to Organize an Information-Support Group for College Students with Hearing Loss

While the development of a college support group for the hearing impaired is not a unique concept (Berg, 1972), ours focused on students who had very good hearing and speech skills and who had "gotten-by" in a normal hearing school environment (Flexer, Wray, & Black, 1986). The first step towards group development focused primarily on expanding the relationship previously established between the **University's Adviser for Handicapped Students** and the University's Speech and Hearing Clinic. The audiology and speech/language clinical supervisors (at the University's Speech and Hearing Clinic) became both advocates and consultants by establishing a **referral system** with the adviser which served to direct new students to our program. To explain: on university application for admission forms, students can choose to state that they have a hearing loss (or any disability). Those applications with stated disabilities are sent to the Adviser for Handicapped Student Services (some universities call this position, "Adviser for Special Student Services"). The advisor then personally saw, called, or wrote to all students who noted that they had a hearing loss, and strongly suggested that they contact the Speech and Hearing Center. We have no idea how many students with hearing loss there are on campus who did not so report on their application forms.

Students voluntarily contacted our center in response to these referrals. In addition, we mailed **personal letters** to all students with hearing loss identified by the Office of Handicapped Student Services explaining the purpose of what became known as "the support-information group for college students who are hard-of-hearing." For many, it was discovered that this group was their first contact with other students with hearing loss receiving education in an integrated setting.

Once the group was formed, our job was to discover the areas of greatest student need which would help to decide the direction of the group. That is, what could the group do to best provide structure and support for the students? What could be done to help the students stay in school, and to have college become a positive educational experience?

Needs of College Students Who Are Hard-of-Hearing

As mentioned in Chapter 1 of this book, the students lacked a great deal of information which could be vital to their success in college. For example, they did not know about basic University support services, conversational coping strategies, hearing aids, assistive listening devices, or even about their own hearing loss. Diedrichsen (1987) points out that this lack is not surprising, given the service delivery system. Even though the vast majority of the twenty million persons with hearing loss in the United States are not "deaf" (no usable hearing, even with amplification), teacher-training programs and rehabilitation training programs focus almost exclusively on the "deaf" population. Therefore, the person with a more moderate hearing loss tends to be treated either as "deaf," or as normally hearing, neither service being suitable (Blair & Berg, 1982; Ross, 1977). As a result, most of these college students had not been appropriately serviced during their school years and arrived at the university with many problems.

For a more specific need definition, a pretest was given verbally to assess:

1. Knowledge of the ear (auditory mechanism)
2. Knowledge of type and degree of their own hearing loss
3. Ability to understand their own audiogram
4. Knowledge of the structure and function of their hearing aid
5. Knowledge of assistive listening devices
6. Awareness of the effect of their hearing loss on communicative interaction.

This group of students has had hearing loss all of their lives and has worn amplification for an average of seventeen years. Nevertheless, the results of this pretest, administered to twenty students, revealed the following information:

Ninety-two percent could not interpret their own audiogram correctly with ten of the twenty not having a notion as to meaning. Approximately 75 percent of the students could not display an understanding of the type and degree of their own hearing loss. In fact, two of the students who had symmetrical hearing losses thought they had one "dead ear." Another student with a mild loss in one ear and a severe hearing loss in the other, referred to herself as being "deaf." Only the earmold, battery, and volume control could be identified by all the students who wore hearing aids. Further, ten of these students could recognize the telecoil switch, but only seven could identify it correctly. Seven had never used their telecoil switch and four of these students reported complete avoidance of the telephone.

None of the students were aware of any assistive listening devices. One student knew about "those bulky auditory trainers," but felt that nothing like that could be appropriate at the university level (Leavitt, 1987).

Audiometric and hearing aid assessments were also performed, and results revealed that not one student had appropriate amplification!! That is, their residual hearing was not maximized, especially through the higher frequencies, with most students having hearing aids which were at least five years old. Specifically, only seven of the twenty had binaural amplification, yet most had essentially symmetrical hearing losses. No one had acoustically modified earmolds, like Libby horns, which would promote better detection of the higher frequencies. Unfortunately, inappropriate amplification tends to be a recurrent problem with this group (Davis, 1977; Davis, Shepard, Stelmachowicz & Gorga, 1981; Flexer & Wray, 1984; Kodman, 1963).

Through discussions at group meetings, lack of knowledge was also shown in the areas of telephone skills, University accommodations, trouble shooting hearing aids, understanding contemporary slang, and use of discourse strategies (Flexer, Wray, & Black, 1986). For example, the students were unaware that they had the right to request that pay telephones with built-in amplifiers be provided for them in college buildings. Further, many of the students did not know basic telephone strategies, such as repeating information and spelling names to be sure that all was understood correctly. In addition, lack of simple hearing aid trouble shooting skills was noted when students brought their hearing aids into the clinic for repair. In three instances, the battery was dead. In another, the earmold was plugged with ear wax.

Language-related semester goals for the group included the introduction of contemporary idioms, and colloquial terms and phrases used by students at the university (e.g., "Let's blow this popsicle stand," "foxy lady," "what a drag," "stay tuned," "pain in the neck," "awesome"). A multiple-choice test, using twenty common idioms, revealed that 70 percent of the students had difficulty recognizing the definition of these concepts. For example, one student thought that a "foxy lady" really looked kind of like a fox (the animal), rather than being very attractive.

It also became obvious that the students had difficulty tuning into the intonation used by a speaker to impart the real meaning of a phrase. Sarcasm is typically conveyed by a twist of stress patterns, rather than by a change of words. For example, when someone says, "I like your hair!", the intended meaning would change depending upon **how** the words are spoken. The speaker could indeed like one's hair, or, depending upon the stress patterns in the speech, he or she could think you look awful! We found that an auditory training approach was necessary to help students learn how to "listen" for those meaningful changes in intonation.

Nonverbal communication skills appeared lacking during conversations. Visual feedback necessary for the listener's benefit was noted to be inappropriate, indifferent, or lacking altogether, making it difficult to determine the level of comprehension and interest in a topic. For example, students tended to nod "yes" even if they did not understand the message. Or, they would stare blankly at the speaker which tended to frustrate both parties of the conversation.

This surprising lack of information about their hearing loss, hearing aids, and effective communication skills was not a result of the students' inability to understand the concepts. Rather, it appeared to be a result of a gap in their previous aural habilitation services, as mentioned in Chapter 1. More importantly, because the students lacked information, they tended to avoid difficult situations and thus to be victimized by, rather than mastering, their hearing loss.

A crucial finding was the lack of preparation for the University curriculum noted in the majority of students with hearing loss. As a result, 75 percent of these students were enrolled in noncredit developmental courses. Specifically, 40 percent took the math developmental course, 60 percent took English developmental courses and 33 percent took both English and math developmental courses. These developmental courses were required as a result of their low scores on entry level tests.

All of the above results indicated that these students displayed a cluster of educational and emotional needs which had to be addressed. Some students needed only minor intervention to succeed. Others would have, quite literally, flunked out of the University without some way to organize support services. Therefore, an information-support group became an important vehicle for facilitating success.

What Does the Group Do?

The needs assessments revealed problem areas mentioned above which then became group goals. The group has been meeting once every other week for almost five years with an average of six to seven students attending every meeting.

The imparting of information about hearing, hearing loss, and audiogram meaning was a primary goal. As previously noted, the students lacked information about their hearing loss. Therefore, students were individually encouraged to develop a simple description of their own hearing loss and how their loss affected communication ability (see Chapter 2). We then role-played how this information could be conveyed in various situations (e.g., during conversation with friends, in discussion with a professor, etc.).

The group also discussed and practiced troubleshooting hearing aids. Many of the students were not comfortable with the daily care of their own hearing aids and were not sure about when to send the aid to the factory

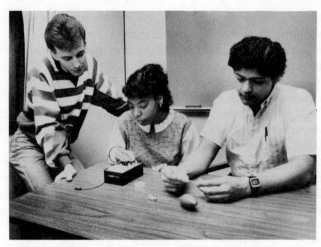

**Figure 13-1: Students Discussed and Practiced Troubleshooting
Hearing Aids.**

for service. Students were taught how to inspect visually their aids for
battery operation, ear wax in the ear molds, cracked ear mold tubing,
broken switches, cracked earhooks, and corroded battery compartments.
In short, the students were empowered to assume responsibility for
their hearing losses and for their hearing aids (Figure 13-1).

*Through ongoing audiometric assessments, attempts were made to update
each student's amplification and to encourage their use of assistive listening
devices (ALD).* This process has taken longer than anticipated due to the
necessity of finding funding for many (see Chapter 7). Also, even though
the University is prepared to loan appropriate assistive listening devices,
students have been reluctant to use them (Leavitt, 1987). Introduction
to new amplification, new earmolds, and new assistive listening devices
has been a gradual process. These are dramatic changes for many of the
students, and we found that we must proceed one step at a time, rather
than attempt to revise completely a student's listening environment all
at once. For example, changing frequency responses of hearing aids
tended to induce anxiety in the students if those changes were substantial. We found that we needed to alter hearing aid frequency responses in small steps to have the changes be acceptable. Further, the
students required practice and proof that ALDs were superior to their
own aids in a classroom environment (Flexer, Wray, Black & Millin,
1987).

*Group language goals involved the development of nonverbal communi-
cation skills, including gestures, facial expressions, and body language.* Dem-
onstrations and role playing were used to show how nonverbal

communication played a significant part in dating and job-interview situations. Idioms and current University slang were also discussed. However, vocabulary difficulties and expressive and receptive language comprehension were dealt with in individual therapy (see Chapter 10).

Role playing was used to practice for job interviews which revolved around career decisions (Menchel, 1984). The students were often uncomfortable in an interview situation and were unsure as to the impact of their hearing loss in certain potential career choices. For example, one student didn't know if her hearing loss would prevent her from entering the nursing program. Another wasn't sure if he could be effective in personnel work. Group discussions helped students problem solve and try to assess the communication demands of different job settings. *In addition, successful persons with hearing loss from the community spoke to the group to function as role models and to provide insight into their own accomplishments. Career counselors from the University also served as guest speakers on this topic* (see Chapter 14).

Social development and campus leisure activities have been other topics addressed through varying group dynamics. Appropriate and acceptable social interaction is so very important for success in the hearing world (Hummel & Schirmer, 1984). Therefore, simulations of dating scenes, telephone contacts, and "how to converse in the noisy student center," were employed. Students also practiced talking about their hearing loss, another very difficult task for them (Spangenberg, 1982).

A particularly enjoyable activity has occurred when we combined the clinic group for parents of children who are hearing impaired with the college group (Flexer & Wray, 1989). The parents stated that they needed to see that their toddlers with hearing loss could grow up to be college students. Further, parents asked the college students probing questions such as, "What do you wish that your parents had or had not done for you as you were growing up?" and "Did you ever not want to wear your hearing aids?" and "When were you able to talk about your hearing loss with your parents?" The college students expressed that this meeting allowed them to be the "experts" while gaining new insights into their own parents' motives.

Summary

It has often been assumed that the student with hearing loss who has been accepted into a university can function independently, requiring no special support services. However, this assumption appears to be false in almost every instance. The purpose of this chapter has been to discuss some of the needs of college students who are hearing impaired, to describe the development of a support group for these students, and to present some group activities.

Because the majority of the students lacked basic knowledge about their own hearing loss, hearing aids, assistive listening devices, University support services, telephone strategies, and contemporary slang, **a primary function of the group was to serve as a clearing house for new information**. No less important were emotional needs. Fortunately, the students stated that the group also provided a support system for them as many had not had previous contacts with other students with hearing loss. **Most important, the group has allowed them to openly acknowledge and discuss their hearing losses, often for the very first time.** Therefore, the support group appears to serve a very important function in helping students with hearing loss succeed in a hearing university.

Checklist of How to Start a College Support Group

1. The Support Group is typically operated out of the university's speech and hearing clinic with audiologists and speech-language pathologists working together.

2. A partnership is established between the university's speech and hearing clinic and the university's Adviser for Handicapped (or Special) Student Services.

3. The audiologist and speech-language pathologist meet with the Adviser to explain the unique needs of students with hearing loss.

4. A referral system is organized whereby the Adviser directs all students with hearing loss to the speech and hearing clinic.

5. Personal letters are mailed and phone calls are made by the speech and hearing clinic to all students who have identified themselves as hearing impaired on their college admission applications.

6. Once some students with hearing loss are interested in organizing and meeting, they, too, can contact prospective members.

7. Try to organize meeting times to be convenient for all, and be flexible.

8. Meeting twice a month might be better than four times a month so as not to interfere with study time.

9. Serving refreshments at meetings helps to generate an informal atmosphere.

Checklist of Activities for the College Support Group

1. Arrange appointments for complete hearing tests and hearing aid assessments.

2. Arrange for use of Assistive Listening Devices (ALD).

3. Provide information about hearing loss, hearing aids, current technology, and about the effects of hearing loss on academic and social performance.

4. Provide information about filling out employment applications and simulate job-interview situations.

5. Have guest speakers addressing career choices, e.g., university career counselors and successful persons with hearing loss from the community.

6. Have an attorney speak about legal issues surrounding hearing impairment, e.g., rights and responsibilities.

7. Have discussions and impart information about telephone strategies, including use in social and employment settings.

8. Discuss and practice current student slang.

9. Discuss difficult social situations, and role play as a problem solving technique.

10. Have the Adviser for Handicapped Student Services speak to the group about the services to which they are entitled.

11. Participate in numerous altruistic activities, including meeting with parents of younger children with hearing loss, meeting with adolescents who are hearing impaired and their parents, and serving as guest speakers in local schools.

References

Berg, F.S. (1972). A model for a facilitative program for hearing impaired college students. The *Volta Review, 74*, 370–375.

Blair, J., & Berg, F. (1982). Problems and needs of hard-of-hearing students. *ASHA, 24*, 541–546.

Davis, J. (1977). Our forgotten children: Hard-of hearing pupils in the schools. In J. Davis (Ed.), *Our Forgotten Children: Hard-of-Hearing Pupils in the Schools*. Minneapolis, MN: National Support Systems Project and Division of Personnel Preparation, Bureau of Education for the Handicapped, Department of Health, Education, and Welfare.

Davis, J.M., Shepard, N.T., Stelmachowicz, P.G. & Gorga, M.P. (1981). Characteristics of hearing impaired children in the public schools: Part two psychoeducational data. *Journal of Speech and Hearing Disorders, 46*, 130–137.

Diedrichsen, R. (1987). Towards the acquisition of basic rights and services for persons who are hard of hearing. *SHHH, 8*(2), 3–4.

Flexer, C., & Wray, D. (1984). Congenitally hearing impaired college students: The forgotten group. *Hearing Instruments, 35,* 20; 49.

Flexer, C., & Wray D. (1989). Role models: Hearing impaired college students reach out to the community. The *Volta Review, 91,* 157–162.

Flexer, C., Wray, D.F., & Black, T.S. (1986). Support group for moderately hearing impaired college students: An expanding awareness. *Volta Review, 88,* 223–229.

Flexer, C., Wray, D., Black, T., & Millin, J. (1987). Amplification devices: Evaluating classroom effectiveness for moderately hearing impaired college students. The *Volta Review, 89,* 347–357.

Hummel, J.W., & Schirmer, B.E. (1984). Review of research and description of programs for the social development of hearing impaired students. The *Volta Review, 86,* 259–266.

Kodman, F. (1963). Educational status of hard of hearing children in the classroom. *Journal of Speech and Hearing Disorders, 28,* 297–299.

Leavitt, R.J. (1987). Promoting the use of rehabilitation technology. *ASHA, 29,* 28–31.

Menchel, R. (1984). Preparation for the world of work. The *Volta Review, 86,* 71–84.

Ross, M. (1977). Definitions and descriptions. *American Annals of the Deaf, 122,* 5–18.

Spangenberg, C.P. (1982). Getting to know you—hearing impaired style. The *Volta Review, 84,* 239–243.

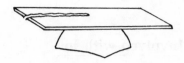

Chapter 14
Is There Anything out There for Me?

Joseph Sendelbaugh, Ed.D., John Freeburg, M.S.

As we look at the title of this chapter "Is There Anything out There for Me?" the answer is happily, "Yes." The range of occupations open to persons with hearing loss is greater than ever before. Surveys conducted throughout the 1980's show very clearly that individuals with hearing impairment are finding employment, and that persons such as your-selves who are continuing their education beyond high school, are in a very favorable position (Bullis, 1985; Schroedel, 1986). Some research has shown that college graduates with hearing impairment can look forward to an open job market (El-Khiami, 1986; Passmore, Marron, Seligman, & Wilson, 1977). In fact, there are successful workers with hearing impairments in all occupational areas and at all levels of repon-sibility and complexity.

The goal of this chapter will be to describe a job-selection process that will help the college student with hearing loss find a training pro-gram that will best fit his or her interests, and in which there appears to be a good likelihood of finding a job after completion of training.

Do I Take the First Job That Pays Well?

If until now you have had only part-time jobs, with pay being the only thing that has been important; and, if you are looking for a job for only a few months, money may be a good selecting tool. Generally, however, college graduates have reported that salary is actually less important than finding a job that matches their personality (Schroedel,

1986). Thus, finding a good match between job responsibility and worker personality is a major focus of this chapter.

How Does My Personality Get Involved with Job Targets?

Generally, in your personal life, you tend to do what you like to do, not what someone else thinks you should do. Your own likes and interests are the most important factors in successful career choices. You need to keep in mind that your career is a reflection of your personality. And remember, you probably will spend one-third of your time, or approximately 80,000 hours on the job, during your working life. So, it would make sense to select an occupation that you will enjoy.

Experience has shown the authors that there are three activities that can give a person insight into his/her personality:

1. hobbies,
2. past memories, and
3. an imaginary "perfect" job.

The types of hobbies you have are a very strong indication of the types of activities that you would probably enjoy in a job. For example, if making scenery is pleasurable, perhaps landscaping or designing may be the field to investigate. Along with hobbies, interest in sports might also give you a clue to your best occupational choice. That is, if you love physical activity, a job that requires sitting behind a desk might not be matched to your interests.

You probably can remember a few events from your early childhood with great detail. Why you remember these particular events is not easily explained, but it does suggest that these events were significant to you. They might also help you to identify characteristics of a good occupational choice. For example, if you enjoyed tutoring other students in high school, perhaps a teaching career might be a satisfying future job.

A third way you can gain some insight into your occupational interest is by using your imagination. In order to let your imagination do its job, begin by assuming that you have all the training or education needed to land any position. Choose the best possible job and then ask yourself the classic "wh" questions about your fantasy: "What" is my job? "Where" are my job and home located? "Whom" am I working with? "When" do I work? This exercise should lead to one or two short paragraphs that you can add to your other list of responses from above.

With your written list of hobbies, past positive experiences, and your imaginary future occupation in hand, you need to write two or three sentences about how each of these ideas are similar. Often very common trends will appear, forming an excellent base on which we can continue our exploration.

Now that I Have Looked at Myself, How Do I Look at Different Jobs?

There are as many ways to classify jobs as there are currently available career books. Basically, the majority of classifications tend to break down jobs into three general types. For example, the *Dictionary of Occupational Titles*, the largest single source of job names, assigns each occupation to one of three areas:

1. **Data**. Jobs that require high levels of "data" skills are those jobs which stress information, investigation, interpretation, numbers, words, symbols, ideas, and concepts. Examples of occupations in this area would include craftsman, scientist, computer operator/ programmer, or mathematician.
2. **People**. Jobs related to people are those which focus heavily on providing counseling, exchanging ideas, teaching, supervising, or serving. Positions that require dealing with animals on an individual basis are also found in this group of jobs. Doctors, veterinarians, counselors, teachers, and salespeople are part of this group.
3. **Things**. Our third area of job classification, "things," centers around working with machines and tools. Positions that require a high degree of interest in things would be truck drivers, mechanics, lumberjacks, tool and die makers, and computer designers.

Our next step in the job selection process is to classify what we learned about ourselves in the last section, according to the three characteristic areas of data, people, and things. At this point, some trends should begin to form. Compare your final two or three summary sentences from the previous section, "your personality," with what you have done in this section, "different jobs." Do they make sense? Hopefully, a consistent picture of your career interests is forming.

Am I Ready to Investigate Job Titles Now?

Since this book is intended for the college student who is also hearing impaired, let's consider the part that hearing loss could play in your early career planning efforts. Based on several studies and the authors' experience, the amount of hearing loss is not the most significant issue (Blewitt, 1976; Phillips, 1975). The ability to understand and discriminate speech is actually more critical to the successful selection of a job. Every work setting or environment has different levels of noise that may interfere with oral communication. Two clerical positions may have the same job description but one may be in a large office with many telephones ringing and computers being used all day, while another position may have only one typist working alone with no telephones. How well could you understand oral instructions or questions in these two situations? Sadly, there are no indexes that rate how noisy a particular job may be. So, if you have any usable hearing, establishing an ideal situation depends on your working closely with a qualified audiologist experienced in assistive listening technology.

How Do I Find out Specific Job Titles in Which I May Be Interested?

At this point you should have a good idea about whether you prefer working with people, data, or things. With this basic information you can use the "government document center" at most large libraries. The Department of Labor produces a great deal of information concerning job requirements and future employment trends. Many of these publications use a six digit code to identify major areas and characteristics of more than "20,000" jobs.

The first three digits of the six-digit job code divide each occupation into a general job family. For example, number "001" would be architectural occupations. The last three digits are connected to our previous work with data, people, and things. Let's look at an example to help you understand this code system.

Example: code 939.387
939.—— indicates occupations dealing with mining of minerals; in our example this is a "coal inspector".
—.3— indicates that the person in this job must compile data.
——.-8- indicates that the job requires no connection with other people, you tend to work alone.
and
——.—7 indicates that you must handle things, or move things on this job.

Particular publications that you should investigate that use this six digit code, and that have a great deal of occupational information, are: *The Occupational Outlook Handbook, Occupational Outlook Handbook in Brief, Occupational Outlook Handbook Quarterly*, and the *Monthly Labor Review*.

In addition, your library will also have other texts. A sample of career reference books that may be helpful would be: *Encyclopedia of Careers and Vocational Guidance, College Placement Annual*, and *Career Guidance to Professional Associations*. The journal and magazine sections will also have various business or money-management publications that will often highlight growing and different professions.

Most of us are unaware of many possible jobs and careers. Did you know about the following job descriptions?:

a. *Surveyors*: establish official land and water boundaries, write descriptions of land for deeds and other legal documents, and collect information for the preparation of maps and charts.

b. *Recreation Workers*: plan, organize, and direct activities that help people enjoy and benefit from leisure hours. May work in community centers, parks, camps, schools, correctional centers, and adult day-care centers.

c. *Dental Lab Technicians*: skilled craft workers who make and repair a wide variety of dental appliances.

d. *Product and Packaging Designers*: arrange and design articles, products, and materials in such a way that they are not only functional, but also visually pleasing.

Since some persons reading this section may already be attending colleges and universities, you should make use of your campus job-placement office. These offices are staffed by professionals trained in career counseling, who often schedule interviews for you with prospective employers. These services are usually free to students, and the staff is generally motivated to provide you with a great deal of personal service. Also, be sure that you do not overlook the services of Vocational Rehabilitation (see Chapter 7), the primary vocational support organization for people with hearing loss seeking employment opportunities.

Even with extensive reading and talking with experienced career counselors, research shows that, especially for persons with hearing impairments, there is really no substitute for experience in helping you to narrow down your career interest areas (Bullis, 1985). If there is a type of job that appears interesting, you can learn a great deal more about it by seeking practicum, internship, or volunteer positions in that field. A potential employee with experience in the chosen field is very attractive to employers.

Is a Résumé Important?

Remember that your resume', a written summary of your background, qualifications, and work history, is the first impression that you make on your future employer. A résumé should be easy to read and generally straightforward. For a person just beginning post-college work experience, a one or two page résumé should be sufficient. Remember that in most cases, many people are applying for the same position, so those who are screening applicants will not spend a great deal of time reading every application. Your résumé should accent your strengths in both school performance and work experience. Most college career placement offices offer guidelines for developing an effective résumé.

What Goes into an Interview?

When you go into a job interview, you should know what the employers are looking for. Of course, most employers are looking for people who have the appropriate training for their open position. In addition, the prospective employee should appear to get along with his peers, and to be interested in continuing his or her education in a particular occupation.

Attempting to hide a disability is viewed as extremely negative. In fact, one reason given by employers as to why they had fired personnel in the past is that when the workers first applied for the position, they hid their physical disabilities which limited their ability to do their work (Phillips, 1975). Federal law does prohibit employers from asking about physical disabilities unless there would be some direct connection to the job; however honesty is generally the best policy. Nevertheless, you need not dwell on the issue of your hearing loss. An acceptable way to handle the question of your hearing loss might be to try to turn it to a positive feature. A response you might give to a question such as "What do you see as your greatest weakness" could be, "My hearing loss may at first glance appear to be a problem, but it has taught me to be a careful listener."

As pointed out earlier, you will need to know how your speech discrimination ability will "fit in" to the work environment. If you can describe in detail how well you can hear in a particular environment, especially with the use of assistive communication technology, you will assure your future employer that your hearing loss is not a barrier to your successful performance.

Now that I Have a Great Job, I Won't Need to Think About Another Job for the Rest of My Life, Right?

The odds of staying on one job for the next forty years are very slim. In the United States, the average worker will change jobs six to seven times in a lifetime. In addition, almost 25 percent of today's jobs will no longer exist forty years from now. Hopefully you have learned a career selection method that will help you to plan your first job and also help you to change jobs in the twenty-first century.

Career Planning Outline

_____ Develop a summary of my past positive experiences based on my interests and my personality (2–3 sentences).

_____ Review books for career selection from the library (example *Occupational Outlook Handbook*).

_____ Write a letter to National Associations in the career areas in which I am interested.

_____ Consult with my high-school guidance counselor or rehabilitation counselor BEFORE selecting an education program, in order to make sure that the program is appropriately accredited.

_____ Consult with an audiologist about my speech discrimination ability in various work environments.

_____ Review with an audiologist the assistive listening devices most appropriate for classroom use and future work environments.

_____ Visit training programs where I can learn about my future career area.

_____ Meet staff of the college's special student services offices. Find out if they have other students with hearing loss in attendance.

_____ Contact my local office of Vocational Rehabilitation and/or the college's financial-aid office to find out about scholarships that may help me pay for school.

_____ Maintain contact with the college's office of disabled student services to help develop the best learning environment while I am in school.

_____ Before my last six months in school, I will contact the college's office of Career Development Placement to start developing a résumé and to begin interviewing for career positions.

References

Blewitt, E. (1976). *The Relationship between Communication Skills of Young Deaf Adults and Their Success in Employment*. Scranton, PA.: Bloomsburg State College.

Bullis, M. (1985). A dilemma: Who and what to teach in career education programs? In M. Bullis & D. Watson (Eds.), *Career Education of Hearing impaired Students: A Review* (pp. 55–75). Little Rock, AR: Research and Training Center on Deafness/Hearing Impaired.

College Placement Annual (1986–87). Bethlehem, PA: College Placement Council.

El-Khiami, A. (1986). Selected characteristics of hearing impaired rehabilitants of general vocational rehabilitation agencies: A socio-demographic profile. In D. Watson, G. Anderson, & M. Taft-Watson (eds.), *Integrating Human Resources, Technology and Systems in Deafness* (pp. 136–144). Silver Springs, MD: American Deafness and Rehabilitation Association.

Hopke, William E. (ed.) (1981). *Encyclopedia of Careers and Vocational Guidance*. Chicago, IL: J.G. Ferguson Publishing Co.

Passmore, D.L., Marron, M., Seligman, J., & Wilson, F.L. (1977). Industries, occupations, and functions entered by a convenience sample of graduates of NTID (Report No. 15), Rochester, NY: Division of Management Services, National Technical Institute of the Deaf.

Phillips, G.B. (1975). An exploration of employer attitudes concerning employment opportunities for deaf people. *Journal of Rehabilitation of the Deaf, 9*(2), 1–9.

Schroedel, J.G. (1986). A national study of the class of 1984 in post-secondary education with implications for rehabilitation. In D. Watson, G. Anderson, & M. Taft-Watson (eds.), *Integrating Human Resources, Technology and Systems in Deafness* (pp. 267–286). Silver Springs, MD.: American Deafness and Rehabilitation Association.

U.S. Dept. of Labor and Bureau of Labor Statistics, (1986). *Occupational Outlook Handbook*. Washington, DC: Government Printing Office.

U.S. Dept. of Labor and Bureau of Labor Statistics, (1918-). *Monthly Labor Review*. Washington, DC: Government Printing Office.

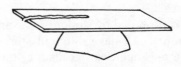

Chapter 15
The Real Experts Speak: Students with Hearing Loss Discuss How to Succeed in College

Susan Coler, Steve Gordon, Kathryn Louden, Doreen McSorley, Peter Paulson, Jenny Schwartzberg, Crystal Terrell, David Viers, and Kim Woods

Introduction

Previous chapters have dealt with topics such as: hearing, hearing aids, vocational rehabilitation, support services, listening devices, academic accommodations, etc. The subject area's diversity reflects the myriad needs of the college student with hearing loss who is competing in a hearing environment.

The authors have attempted to address comprehensively the potential needs of students with hearing loss entering the ranks of higher education. However, the editors would be remiss if they had not invited contributions from the real "experts"—those actually working in the "trenches" of college life. Consequently, this chapter is entirely composed by students with hearing loss who have dared to venture beyond secondary schooling. They deserve commendation for their effort, gratitude for their positive role-modeling, admiration for their tenacity, and an opportunity to share their experiences.

The chapter is a series of writings contributed by students who are hearing impaired from around the country. All have different stories and recommendations to share, but the message clearly calls for other students with hearing loss to continue to carry the torch into hearing universities throughout the country. In some respects, it is the higher-education experience that is the epitome of normalization for these individuals. Equipped with higher educational skills, the student with hearing loss can achieve the dream of becoming a contributing citizen in our society; recognized for skill and ability rather than a disability that is but a small part of the total person.

Making the Choice to Live in a Hearing World

Susan Coler

Every now and then people will be making choices that will affect their lives and change their way of thinking about certain issues. Some choices that individuals make will turn out, while others do not turn out so well. One choice that I made in my life was well worth choosing. It began when I was small, starting out in kindergarten. The school system discovered that I had a severe hearing loss and wanted to place me in the class for students who were mentally retarded at a county school. When my dad found out what the school system had in mind, he had a fit. That's when he fought with the school system to keep me in public school and be mainstreamed. It was my dad who helped me to make the choice of being mainstreamed in a regular classroom.

The war raged on until I was in sixth grade, and that was when the school system stopped fighting with my father and other supporters that I gained throughout my struggle. The school system finally realized that I was able to handle the rigors of a regular classroom. I also proved to them that I had made the choice of wanting to be mainstreamed. It was the best choice that I made in my life.

Today, I am now attending a hearing university that provides assistance for students who are hard-of-hearing and for students with other disabilities. This was a result of my choice of wanting to remain in the regular classroom. After I chose to go to a hearing college, I checked out the services that were available such as tutoring, hearing aid assessments, and free hearing tests for students who are hard-of-hearing. One thing that I took full advantage of was the service of a support group at The University of Akron. The group has helped me tremendously. It showed me one thing—that I'm not the only one with a hearing loss. Once I understood that I was not alone in the world with a hearing loss, that was the one thing that helped me through college. The group also provided information about the services that were available on campus and where to find them. It also provided a medium for making friends.

College life for me is no different than that of a student with normal hearing. I am just like any other person going to college. It is hard and a lot of work. But it is up to the student who is hard-of-hearing whether or not he or she chooses to go to college, or finds out what services are available and if a support group exists on campus. Good luck in college. You *can* make it!

Learning to Cope with Hearing Loss
Steve Gordon

I do not remember when I could hear! My earliest recollections are of battles in trying to understand people's speech. However, I developed my own coping skills distinctive to my condition at an early age.

When I began school, I could cope with the work and I loved reading. My parents already knew that I had a moderate to severe sensorineural hearing loss of an unknown origin and that it was permanent and progressive.

I can remember being nervous and frustrated from the strain of having to construe faint sound patterns, lip reading, and body movements. No one seemed to comprehend my predicament. When I mentioned my distress to the people around me, they didn't seem to care. Because I appeared to cope so well, no one realized my problem. Asking others to repeat or rephrase what they said seemed to annoy them. Motivated by a wish to be accepted, I only said "pardon me" or "huh" when it was necessary.

I never really understood my teachers in school. Most of them appeared frustrated when I did not follow the instructions in class. I learned to cope by reading directions meticulously and asking other students what the teacher had said or by looking at other classmates' notes.

During my teenage years, I was taken to numerous hearing specialists for testings and re-evaluations. They all said precisely the same thing. From their diagnoses, nothing could be done except to continue wearing my hearing aid and to look for a newer and stronger aid. I sensed many times that none of the doctors wanted to deal with the psychological aspect of my disability; they offered nothing of practical, realistic value to me in my developmental years.

College began for me as a nightmare of hardship, frustration, and apprehension. After all, I was thirty-six years old. I had lost my job and remembered how hard it was for me to learn in my earlier years. I wondered if it would be any better or worse some eighteen years later. My fears were well founded, for nothing had changed. My first semester was difficult because the classroom was next to the main highway and the noise was overwhelming. The second classroom was much the same until one teacher, Mrs. Questel, notified Beth Olmstead, Director of Student Services for the Handicapped. She contacted me at home and told me to meet with Dr. Denise Wray at The University of Akron Speech and Hearing Center, Department of Communicative Disorders.

It was in Dr. Wray's office that I poured out my frustrations of trying to hear and learn in school. For this I am grateful. She introduced me to other staff members who not only worked there, but took me seriously and respected me. With the help of these people, Shuvawn Sweet, Sharon Cargill, Kim McCarthy, Susan Davis, Dr. Carol Flexer, and others too numerous to mention but equally important to me, we talked, tried different hearing aids, and experimented with different assistive listening devices. I never sensed any impatience, but a great deal of interest and concern. I was informed that the University clinic had a support group for students with hearing loss that might be able to help me. Little did I know that these meetings were going to change my life. Through the support group, I came to know Sharon, Crystal, Ned, Helen, Jim, and others. Although all younger than I, all had or were having the same problems in school as I had. We came together every two weeks to share our problems and to listen and suggest possible solutions. It was during one of these meetings that I started to see myself as a unique and special person, as rare as each person around me. I discovered that in order to cope with the hearing world, I had to change many of the old patterns I had established during the years since high school, and to develop the skills needed to deal appropriately with various people and situations. At times I didn't believe in my ability to handle these problems, but the continued support of the group, gave me encouragement, faith, companionship, cheer, and humor.

Students and parents must form support groups or visit a counselor. They must face what they are, hearing impaired, or the parents of a child who is hearing impaired. They must acknowledge their disability to others with pride and dignity. Nobody is going to understand your problem if you don't tell them.

Parents and educators must be more sensitive to the needs of students who are hearing impaired. They must be willing to wear the microphone of an FM assistive listening device and provide another student to take notes. Parents are going to have to be more determined in seeking the kind of help that is available for their children. There are many state and local organizations such as the United Way or national organizations such as Self-Help for Hard of Hearing People Inc., (Shhh for short).

In my meetings with the support group, I have met parents who say their spouse refuses to acknowledge that their child has a hearing loss. Support groups provide encouragement. You do not know of the loneliness and despair we go through when we cannot hear the things that you do. Persons who are hearing impaired, in most cases, even with a listening device, cannot hear the sound of a chirping bird, church bells, or some musical instruments. We are not putting on an act for attention when we say we cannot hear something; after all, how would you know?

For medical-related professions, whether it be a psychologist, audiologist, otolaryngologist, or speech-language clinician, it is imperative that you become more aware of other sources of help including new technology and equipment, such as sound systems and signaling devices. If you cannot afford these pieces of equipment, at least write to the manufacturer and ask for suggested literature or pamphlets to pass out. The medical profession must also become aware of the psychological and sociological problems that people with hearing loss must face. Among them are the dread of crowds, strained telephone use, problems at meetings, and inadequate sound systems at theaters.

Finally, to the person who is hearing impaired. Let your disability be a challenge to you. Get involved in organizations that support your needs. Speak out about your condition, explain to others the best you can what it is like to experience hearing loss. Be proud that you are a special person with a special problem. There will be setbacks and defeats, but it's not the end.

I hope you notice throughout this article the words *hearing impaired*. I never mentioned the word *deaf*. That's because there is already too much emphasis placed on the needs of people who are deaf and not nearly enough on the needs of the people who are functionally hard-of-hearing. Although we are like people who are deaf, we are different in that we have learned to use our remaining hearing to a greater extent. Hopefully, this passage will help address some of the specific needs of people who are hard-of-hearing.

Reflections on a Unilateral Hearing Loss

Kathryn Louden

I am twenty-three years old, a terrible athlete, a good cook, blue-eyed, brown-haired, the youngest of eight children, and a graduate student studying audiology.

I also happen to be profoundly deaf in my left ear, while the hearing in my right ear is fine. This type of loss is called unilateral or "one sided" loss. I wear CROS hearing aids which take the sound that should be heard by my left ear and transfer it over into the right ear so that I can hear it. I purchased the CROS aid just three years ago.

Okay, so I don't have hearing in one ear. I should still be able to function all right because I have normal hearing in the other ear, right? Wrong! If you were to meet me on the street and I wasn't wearing my hearing aids you would probably never guess that I'm hearing impaired. I could carry on a normal conversation and you'd walk away without giving my communication status a second thought. If you were to meet me at a party or some place with a lot of noise in the background you'd probably find me sticking close to someone I know and I'd be reluctant to talk to you. You'd walk away from this situation thinking I was very shy, but a hearing impairment probably wouldn't cross your mind. Having a unilateral hearing impairment alters your ability to communicate with people. I can't participate in one-to-one conversations with a lot of noise in the background. I often can't tell where a sound is coming from. I can't always communicate effectively even when I'm in a one-to-one situation. I have all of my close friends and family trained to walk on my right side (my hearing side) to help avoid this problem. Sometimes I can hear what's being said to me, but I can't understand it. It sounds muffled and distant.

I once had a doctor tell me that my hearing impairment could be compared to a glass of water that's half full. I could either look at the glass as half full and take on a positive attitude concerning my disability and learn to deal with it on my own, or look at the glass as half empty and have a negative view of my hearing loss. I don't think I have a negative attitude about my impairment, but when my glass is half empty and everyone else's is full I'm going to need help. I need help in classroom situations. Preferential seating is a fantasy. While it's better to sit near the speaker than in the back of the room, it's not the "be all and end all" of resources that a teacher has available to them. I need help in movie theaters or other public places where assistive listening devices could be used. I need my otologist or even my family physician to keep up to date on what can be done for people with hearing loss, and keep me informed. I need for my friends and family to learn communication strategies that will help when we converse. It may sound like I'm asking a lot, but it's really not much when you can consider the end results—a half empty glass that works almost as well as a full one!

Capitalizing on Accommodations Available in College

Doreen McSorely

Success in college is difficult for anyone. It takes hard work and dedication. A person with a hearing impairment has more difficulty succeeding in college. My own experience has taught me that you have to be persistent and stand up for your rights. You also need to learn about hearing loss and available technology. You should also consider joining or forming a group for students with hearing loss.

Before you start college, you need some basic information. First you need to learn about your legal rights as a person who is hard-of-hearing. Public colleges and universities receive federal funding and are required by law to provide a full range of auxiliary aid options including: qualified sign interpreters, TTY/TDD, supplemental hearing devices such as those described in Chapter 5, flash cards, and notetakers. You have the right to request these devices or aids to gain access to classes and even for entertainment purposes. For example, college and university plays and concerts must be accessible to students who are hard-of-hearing.

My first experience in college was frustrating. I went to the Disabled Student Services on the campus and told them I was a student who was hearing impaired. Their reaction was, "What do you want us to do for you?" I had no idea what my rights were or what services might benefit me. They would not or possibly could not tell me what was available. As a result, I received no services. I struggled for four-and-a-half years trying to take notes in my classes. When I missed something, I would try to get notes from someone else. This made me too dependent on other people and I did not like it. When I started my master's program at Oregon State College as a teacher of students who are hearing impaired, I found out that college does not have to be frustrating. The Disabled Student Services at Western, as it's called, had people that cared and were willing to help. I received a notetaker and they informed me of their other services. They have also loaned me a personal FM system to use in my classes.

In addition to learning about your legal rights and available services, you also should learn about technology for people with hearing loss. The first piece of technology that I found out about was my hearing aid. I wore my hearing aid for five years before I knew anything about it, except how to turn it on and off, change the battery, and adjust the volume. I had no idea of how the hearing aid worked or how to perform routine maintenance. The second technology I learned about was a personal FM system. Having a personal FM system has made attending classes less frustrating. I can now listen to the professor without the distraction of background noise. The third kind of technology I learned about was the loop system to listen to movies, musical performances, television, stereos, and lectures. I can hear much clearer using a loop than I ever dreamed was possible.

As I said before, when you begin college, you also need to have a support group of some type. At Western, students with hearing loss have a club. We hold weekly meetings, put on dances, and present free closed-captioned movies twice a month. We also serve as a support system for each other. It's great to know there are other people who are going through the same types of experiences that I do. There is always someone to talk to, or just listen. I have never had that before. My parents tried to understand my hearing loss and the problems it created, but they really could not.

Being a member of this student club also helped me learn how to be a self-advocate. I have done some public speaking. That is something I never thought I would have the courage to do. I also learned how to accept my hearing impairment. It's all right to be hearing impaired. You should not let your hearing loss stop you from doing the things that you want to do.

Progress on All Fronts

Peter J. Paulson, D.D.S.

I was raised and educated in Minneapolis, Minnesota, with Dr. Win Northcott as my first teacher. Born with a severe to profound hearing loss as a result of the rubella epidemic of 1964, my parents and I were enrolled in the family-oriented oral preschool program at the Minneapolis Hearing Society, of which Win was the Director. I was three years old, at the time. Later I began my formal oral education in special classes and from third grade on I was in regular classes ("mainstreamed" or "integrated") in the public schools of Minneapolis.

I wear binaural hearing aids, first fitted when the diagnosis of hearing loss was established, and rely primarily on speech reading for acquisition of information and conversation in everyday living. My hearing aids are useful in supplying supplemental information about the noise in my environment; a general knowledge of the source of sound, and an awareness of pitch and intonation in some people's voices. I cannot understand connected speech and language by hearing alone. My speech is clear and intelligible and I am told I am a superior speech-reader.

Having been life-long friends, Win introduced me to the world of oral interpreting for which I have been grateful ever since. I attended Concordia College in Moorhead, Minnesota and graduated with a B.A. in Biology in 1982, without any oral interpreting service being available. It wasn't an easy four years, relying only on what I could understand through lipreading my professors. They often paced as they spoke or lectured from notes with head often lowered or turned toward the blackboard as they wrote. I had entertained the thought of training friends to interpret for me, but it was too time-consuming for the kind of work load I already had. I was fortunate, though, to have support from true friends and close contact with the faculty at this small college. On the other hand, having graduated from the School of Dentistry at The University of Minnesota in 1988 with a Doctor of Dental Surgery (DDS) degree, it seems almost unthinkable now to have gone through my undergraduate years without an oral interpreter.

Dental school was a somewhat different setting than that of an undergraduate college. Our class was always together, often in the same lecture hall. Since most of our courses ran more than one quarter in length, new classes with different professors were a common pattern. Candy Baggeroer, my oral interpreter, and I drafted a form letter which was sent out on the letterhead of the Office for Students with Disabilities at The University of Minnesota. Each new professor received letters ahead of time explaining my use of an oral interpreter and what to expect of each of us. Thus the professors who lectured were usually aware of my needs in the classroom such as dimming the lights for easier lipreading during slide presentations, instead of turning them off. I didn't feel compelled to watch the speaker's lips all the time because of the huge amount of slide viewing and watching the oral interpreter as well. I occasionally took notes myself to keep major points fresh in my mind.

I also depended on the "Notetaker's Club" to which 90 percent of my class paid a quarterly membership fee and took turns typing notes and xeroxing copies for other members which were shared through a distribution pool. Instead of typing notes when it was my turn, I helped with the tape recordings daily.

The University of Minnesota provided other professionally trained oral interpreters beside Candy Baggeroer, which was a good sign that oral interpreting has been more widely embraced as a critical tool in learning for some students with hearing loss. I would have otherwise missed key words or phrases that would be tested during final exams.

A word of advice for those about to enter college or a professional school: Try to find an oral interpreter you are comfortable with, and communicate any problems you may have so that you can get 100 percent out of the lectures. I probably will continue to use oral interpreters for many more years. At present, I am completing a one-year Advance General Dentistry residency program. I still use oral interpreters for weekly seminars and discussion groups. I am now currently in private practice in Minneapolis.

In closing, I hope this testimony answers some of the questions you may have about oral interpreters. Even though it took some time for the class and me to get used to having such a service in the classroom, it has proved to be a very positive experience all around.

A Staunch Advocate and Consumer of Oral Interpreting

Jenny Schwartzberg

Hello, I'm Jenny Schwartzberg, and I'm an oral (verbal) person who was prenatally deafened due to the rubella epidemic of 1964. I entered Princeton University in the fall of 1983 after a successful career in very good private elementary and secondary schools, where I was the first and only student who was deaf. At Princeton, there had been another student who was deaf who graduated some years ago, so the administration had some experience with my potential problems and offered to pay students to take notes for me. I used such notetakers all the way through my years at Princeton, but swiftly discovered that notes were not enough. I resorted to taking tape recordings of my classes but even though I eventually set up a relatively fast system of student transcription, I generally got them back three days after the class; by that time, I had forgotten what had been said that day. I had experienced the wonderful benefit of oral interpreters at conventions of the Alexander Graham Bell Association for the Deaf, but I needed interpreters almost every day of the week and on short notice for unanticipated lectures.

At the 1984 A.G. Bell convention in Portland, Oregon, I talked to Mark Stern, then a student at Stanford University in California. He had set up a successful program for students on campus to train as oral interpreters at the paraprofessional level. I continued to use tapes and notetakers but became increasingly dissatisfied with them. Returning to Princeton that fall, I pressed the assistant dean of students to implement such a program on campus. She talked to her counterpart at Stanford who had organized the training program there, and convinced the Princeton administration to finance a comparable program for me. One of my friends, Dr. Joseph Rosenstein, had offered to conduct the workshop which was very fortunate, as Joe can be regarded as the "oral interpreter's interpreter." He is known nationally for his professional skills and the quality of his workshops throughout the country.

In the end, it was September of 1985, the fall semester of my junior year, before the first of Princeton's workshops was held during a weekend before students formed other time commitments. An ad placed in the student newspaper drew a substantial sign-up scheduled to begin Friday morning. Hurricane Gloria struck that day, electricity was knocked out, and all classes were canceled. In the end, the workshop was telescoped into two days and the implementation went smoothly.

I attended all sessions and listened with fascination as Joe taught the students about deafness, oral interpreting, and the responsibilities and the challenges of being an interpreter. I provided feedback on how well the students performed and helped to "weed out" those who, through speech defects or foreign accents, were unable to function effectively as interpreters. Five of the students attained a skill level to begin applying their new techniques and knowledge immediately; I provided additional practice for five more on an informal basis during the following weeks. Thus, six interpreters were a great boon to me in classes during the entire semester. The University paid them six or seven dollars an hour, although I suspect some preferred to remain as volunteers. I also want to say that my interpreters have become good friends of mine. I graduated from Princeton in 1988 and I am currently Assistant to the Curator of Rare Books at the Newberry Library, Chicago

Positive Thinking Equals Success in College
Crystal Terrell

I was born in Akron, Ohio. I graduated from East High School in 1985. I have a hearing loss which is severe in my left ear and profound in my right ear. I wear an Oticon hearing aid in my left ear. My hearing aid would not help in my right ear. When I was approximately two, my parents realized that I did not respond to them when they clapped their hands. They took me to the doctor, and he said I had a hearing loss in both ears. My parents took me to an elementary school where they had a special education class for children who are hearing impaired. My teacher also sent me to the regular classroom. After I graduated from high school, my hearing aid dealer referred me to the Bureau of Vocational Rehabilitation Center (BVR). The BVR helped me with college expenses. They helped me a lot. In addition, they assisted in finding me employment.

I am now a sophomore at The University of Akron, majoring in Office Services Technology. Miss Olmstead, Director of the University's Handicapped Student Services, advised me about some of the new services that would help me in the classroom. Everyday I use the FM system called a Comtek in the classroom so that I can hear better and understand what is going on. I also have a notetaker. A notetaker is a person who takes some good notes just in case I miss some important information. If my notetaker is absent, I ask if anyone would be willing to take notes for me. Usually someone will take notes for me. My classmates are very cooperative. My adviser gives me a package of carbonized paper, and I give it to my notetaker. If I get stuck on my homework and need some help, I usually go to my adviser. My adviser will get me a tutor for any subjects that I am having trouble in.

Every other week, we usually have a college support group meeting for college students who are hearing impaired. During our support group, we discuss about what it is like to be hearing impaired, why people treat us differently, how we can explain to people with normal hearing about our hearing aids, FM systems, amplifiers on the phone, etc., and how they work.

When I go to the Speech and Hearing Center at West Hall, I ask someone to check my hearing aid to see if it is working properly. They also provide speech and language therapy, and students with hearing loss usually come in to work on individual sounds or improve language skills. I have taken advantage of both speech and language therapy services.

Recommendations from a Student Having an Acquired Hearing Loss

David Viers

Although I am not an "expert" in hearing impairment, I have had some experience with different people who experience hearing loss, and I have discovered that they are just that—different. They are different from students with normal hearing, and they are different from one another. The degree of loss, the age at which the loss occurred, the personality and history of each person—all these factors will greatly affect that person's future experiences and perceptions. With that in mind, my "story" is obviously a very individual and limited one.

I am presently forty-two years old; my hearing loss is at the border between severe and profound (I have an "average" loss in each ear of over eighty decibels). I grew up with no noticeable hearing loss; the majority of the hearing loss occurred between the ages of thirty-two and thirty-eight.

I received a Bachelor of Science degree in Biology from The University of Pittsburgh when I was twenty-one years old. What is noteworthy about this is that a great amount of my education was acquired before any apparent hearing loss. Consequently, because I have a proven track-record of success in learning, perhaps I have a greater degree of confidence in my ability to master difficult material than the average student who is hearing impaired.

Because I enjoy learning, I have continued taking college-level courses. It has been an interesting experience because of the challenges posed by my hearing loss. I have formulated certain "rules" that I have found helpful in attending college:

1. Let the instructor know immediately that you have a hearing loss.
2. Sit as close to the instructor as possible.
3. Recognize that, if you expect to learn, you *must* be willing to draw attention to yourself. For example, I suggest the following:
   a) If you did not understand the instructor, then ask for a repetition.
   b) It may be necessary for the instructor to phrase the misunderstood statement in a different way.
   c) You may even have to ask the instructor to write certain words on the chalkboard in order for you to understand.
4. It will be necessary for the instructor to repeat questions/statements that your classmates have said.
5. The more information that your instructor can give you in writing, the better.
6. It is very important that you keep up with your assignments and learn as much as you possibly can from your books.
7. If at all possible, you should try to avoid taking classes from instructors that have speech patterns or characteristics that make speech difficult to understand (accents, *unclear* enunciation, a lot of facial hair, etc.)

Within the last year, I have taken several classes that have had some type of sound-enhancement (an Induction Loop system and an FM system). I have added several additional effective communication "rules" to my original suggestions:

1. These sound enhancement systems described in Chapter 5 are wonderful!! Insist on their use in the classroom and other college-sponsored activities. I have found the Loop system to be most beneficial, because:
   a) Multiple microphones can be used in the classroom which removes some of the burden from the instructor in terms of re-

peating questions/comments from your classmates (you *will* have to remind them to use "their" microphones).

b) There is not likely to be any static or interference with a Loop system (that *is* a problem with the FM systems I have used).

c) On the other hand, depending on the building's structure, it is possible to visit the restroom while wearing an FM system during the instructor's lecturing and never miss a word.

2. I feel it is mandatory for the student with hearing loss to have a good "T" switch on the hearing aids. It is possible to do without one, but it is less efficient.

3. When movies, videos, or "talking" slide presentations are used, there will be problems. Just putting the microphone up to the "speaker" will *not* automatically solve the problem. If possible, the video should be captioned, or a direct line used from the video to the amplifier of the Loop system.

4. It is important that the student with hearing loss recognize that, while the sound-enhancement system will greatly improve things, it will still be necessary for this person to assert him/herself on occasion. There will be times when:

a) The system is not working. The instructor should be informed immediately.

b) Your classmates will need to have their statements repeated by the instructor or they will have to be reminded to use the microphones (with the Loop system).

In conclusion, it is important to realize that the student who is hearing impaired will have some difficulties. However, with consideration from classmates and instructors, the learning experience will be a richly rewarding one.

Suggestions for Survival in Higher Education

Kim Woods

For me as a mainstreamed student who is hard-of-hearing, going to elementary, junior high and high school for twelve years was like traveling an arduous road on a rugged terrain. But the beginning of living a college life-style was like climbing a mountain. During my search for the other side, I have crossed many fords and streams. Looking back at my experiences, I recognize a pattern of progressive stages through which a student with hearing loss can learn to survive college.

First, one must realize that being alone and bewildered in a strange environment of unfamiliar faces and new surroundings is quite common both for students with normal hearing and for students with hearing loss. Throughout the first year, there was an excellent opportunity for me to get reacquainted with myself and to learn to express the real me. This beginning step is called accepting and liking myself, which is often the hardest step to climb. When problems do arise, I encourage touching base with home where family and friends offer their loving support. Do not compare yourself with other students. How can you like other people if you cannot like yourself? Think of good reasons why you can offer friendship to others.

Once I felt more at ease with the person inside of me, the next thing I did was to set goals. The only way I achieved them was that I set them within my grasp, so it was easier for me to reach them. Once I reached a goal, I made a new one and set it a little higher, like the next rung of a ladder. However, there were times when I would slip to a lower rung. Frustrating as those times were, I had to keep saying to myself that everyone has her own limitations. I'd have to use an alternative way or make a sacrifice to work around my weaknesses. I suffered embarrassment wearing hearing aids, because benefiting from the sound amplification was far more important than worrying about their appearance. I often had to spend extra hours reading books to make up for the missed key information from lectures. I had to remember not to push myself too hard, for fear I would experience a burnout. On the other hand, I sometimes took necessary risks to face up to a challenge to get ahead and onto the next goal.

To help me along the way, listing my own self needs, whether they were educational or psychological, was the next step. If a college offers any type of services for the student, there should be no hesitancy to use them. Why else are they available?

This idea transfers to the last step. Once a handful of students gather around, they can informally set up a support group. Each person not only gains a new identity of belongingness, but also discovers refreshing insights into dealing with comparable problems once thought to be felt by no one else. To sustain the group's uniformity, everyone must be working together as a team, encouraging one another, and most importantly, communicating well with each other.

As a support group, people with hearing loss can create a powerful voice in the public. We need to shed some light on our disability since it is the most hidden of all disabilities. We can inform a variety of people on campus: the faculty, the students, the administration members, and other members of the staff.

The growing of the support group should not stop here. We can broaden our horizons beyond the campus boundaries to the communities. I, at one particular time, was involved in a presentation put on by myself and three of my friends with hearing loss at a grade school in a small neighboring town by the campus. This presentation, based on our early educational experiences, was especially set up for a fourth-grade girl who had just lost a considerable portion of her hearing. As we reminisced about our past, I will never forget the expression of awe and elation on her little face. This impression led me to think of the future generations and the difference we as college students with hearing loss could make if we can push ourselves beyond our limits. We must be willing to take these steps on the road to success through college to the life beyond.

Summary

It is interesting to note that the students contributing to this chapter were given limited direction about what to include in their writings. Nor were they provided the opportunity of seeing how other students were approaching the task. They were simply requested to make recommendations and/or to include advice and impressions for other students with hearing loss. Their vignettes are poignant and valuable guides. One common trend surfaces: use the services that are available. Do not wait until failure occurs. As students who are hearing impaired, you are entitled to accommodations; therefore use them. Do not rely on the fact that no services may have been necessary in high school. You are no longer in high school. College is a different environment entirely and needs to be approached with a certain amount of educated preparation. It is the wise and successful college student with hearing loss who comes to this realization.

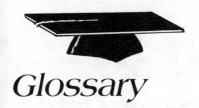

Glossary

Accommodations: Services or equipment to which the student with a disability is legally entitled for the purpose of providing an adequate and equitable education in the learning and working environments.

Accreditation: A process by which a post-secondary (after high school) educational or training institution meets standards of quality for its faculty and program of studies.

Acoustic: This refers to the sense of hearing.

Acoustically Modified Earmolds: Specifically shaped earmolds that change the output of the hearing aid (e.g., "Libby Horn," which improves high frequency amplification).

ACT: The American College Tests are standardized tests used by many colleges and universities as part of their undergraduate admissions testing program.

Aided Thresholds: The softest tones that a person can hear while wearing his/her hearing aids. They are represented by the symbol "A" on the audiogram.

Air Conduction: Sound travels through the air from a source, reaches the ear, enters the auditory system through the ear canal, progresses through the eardrum, middle ear, inner ear and finally to the brain.

Amplification: To make sounds louder. May also refer to a piece of equipment used to make sounds louder, such as a hearing aid.

Assistive Listening Device (ALD): Any of a number of pieces of equipment used to assist the hearing aid in difficult listening situations; provides a superior signal-to-noise ratio.

Audibility: Being able to hear, but not necessarily to distinguish among speech sounds.

Audiogram: A graph of a person's hearing loss, showing both loudness (intensity) and pitch (frequency).

Audiologist: A certified individual with a graduate degree in the assessment and nonmedical management of hearing loss.

Aural Rehabilitation: A series of procedures to help persons deal with their hearing losses, including: use of hearing aids and assistive listening devices, counseling, providing information, improving listening skills, lipreading, speech/language therapy, etc.

Automatic Gain Control (AGC): Conventional amplifiers limit output level by "clipping of peaks" of strong sounds. If this clipping is extreme, significant distortion results. AGC hearing aids limit output levels using a feedback circuit which reduces the gain of the aid when high sound levels are encountered. AGC hearing aids may be useful when the user has a low tolerance level for loud sounds or when there is a narrow range between the faintest sound the user can hear and the loudest sound that can be tolerated.

Basic Hearing Test Battery: The collection of tests given to an individual who wants his/her hearing evaluated, typically including: case history, tuning forks, speech tests (threshold and word identification), pure tone air and bone conduction testing, immittance, and counseling.

Basic Skills Courses: Preparatory courses in reading, writing, and math offered by colleges to help students overcome academic weaknesses in these basic skills.

Behind-the-Ear Hearing Aid: A type of hearing aid which fits over the outer ear so as to be behind the ear of the wearer.

Binaural (hearing aids): The use of two separate hearing aids, one for each ear. Such an arrangement is typically recommended rather than a single hearing aid.

Bone Conduction: A pathway by which sound directly reaches the inner ear through skull vibration, thereby bypassing the outer and middle ear.

Bone Oscillator: The piece of equipment used in bone conduction testing which looks like a small black box attached to a headband.

Bureau of Vocational Rehabilitation: The Bureau of Vocational Rehabilitation (BVR) is a service bureau of the Rehabilitation Services Commission, a state agency responsible for the rehabilitation of the state's physically, mentally, and emotionally disabled citizens. BVR's goal is to aid the disabled person in becoming gainfully employed or as self-sufficient as possible.

Central Auditory Mechanism: That part of the ear structure which includes the brainstem and cortex (brain). Sound is perceived or understood here.

Central "Hearing Loss": Not really a hearing loss in terms of loss of reception, but rather difficulty with the perception or understanding of incoming sounds. The source of the problem is in the brainstem or brain, not in the outer, middle, or inner ear.

Cognitive Overload: The condition of your brain when it has too much to do. Usually, the overloaded brain quietly steps out at important times, leaving you to go on without it temporarily. At these times you make horrible mistakes, or "no-brainers."

College Preparatory Coursework: Taking the appropriate high-school courses which would permit a student to be admitted to college.

Colloquial Terms: Words or phrases used in informal, daily conversation. Phrases which are used or understood in one geographic area may not be used or understood in others (e.g., "ya'll," "yous guys," "you'uns").

Conductive Hearing Loss: A hearing loss caused by damage or disease (pathology) located in the outer or middle ear that interferes with the efficient conduction of sound into the inner ear.

Conductive Mechanism: That part of the ear structure which includes the outer and middle ear.

Congenital Hearing Loss: A hearing loss which begins in the prespeech period; usually refers to a hearing loss that was present at birth.

Conversational Coping Strategies: Techniques used by both the speaker and listener when misunderstandings of the message occur; including repetition of the message, substitutions of different words, or adding new information. All of these techniques serve to improve the understanding of the message.

Cooperative Education: A formal educational program which combines class-room study with on-the-job experience in a paid, academically-related employment position. (All colleges do not have this type of program.)

Coupled: This refers to the connecting or attaching of one object to another, for example, a hearing aid to an assistive listening device.

Credit Hour: A unit used by institutions of higher education to measure/record academic work successfully completed by students.

Degree Granting College: A college that bestows a title that attests to satisfactory completion of specific courses of study.

Developmental Courses: As a result of low scores obtained on college entrance examinations, some students need to take noncredit courses to prepare them to compete in regular freshman-level coursework.

Disability: Impairment or loss of function of whole or parts of body systems.

Distance Hearing: The ability to "overhear" conversations and monitor environmental events . . . an ability which is severely reduced by hearing loss.

Earmold: That part of a hearing aid or ALD which fits in the individual's ear and serves to conduct the sound from the hearing aid into the ear. In-the-ear and in-the-canal hearing aids are usually housed inside the earmold.

Endogenous Hearing Loss: A hearing loss, caused by genetic factors, which could be hereditary (passed on to children or grandchildren).

Exogenous Hearing Loss: A hearing loss which was caused by environmental factors, like a virus or medications, and can therefore not be passed on to children.

Feedback, Acoustic: If too much amplified sound leaks out of the ear and is re-amplified by the hearing aid, a squealing sound (feedback) results. Feedback may happen if the earmold fits poorly, is poorly designed, or not inserted completely. Any situation which reflects sound back into the hearing aid, such as cupping the hand over the aid or standing close to a hard reflective surface, may also cause feedback.

Frequency: Also called pitch and measured in Hz along the top of an audiogram.

Frequency Response: The way that each hearing aid or ALD shapes the incoming (speech) sounds to best reach the individual's hearing loss. It is the amount of amplification provided by the hearing aid at any frequency.

Functional Hearing Loss: Not a real hearing loss, but one which is faked or exaggerated.

Gain: The amount by which the output level of the hearing aid exceeds the input level, or, in simpler terms, how much "louder" sounds are made by the hearing aid.

Hearing Aids: Individual amplification which functions like a miniature public address system to amplify (make louder) and shape the incoming (speech) sounds.

Hearing Aid Stethoscope: An instrument which allows one to listen to the output of a hearing aid in order to detect malfunction.

Horn, Acoustic (of an earmold): Progressive increase of the internal diameter of the earmold sound channel resulting in a "horn effect" which enhances certain sounds. A common use is to restore some of the sound energy associated with ear canal resonance which may be lost when a conventional earmold is inserted into the ear.

Idioms: The assignment of a new meaning to a group of words that already have their own meaning, with the literal meaning no longer serving as the proper interpretation. For example, "a pain in the neck" does not mean that the person is physically ill, but rather that the person is bothersome to another.

Immittance Testing: An objective measure of middle ear function, not hearing sensitivity; measures how well the ear drum moves.

Inner Ear: Comprised of the cochlea (which contains the thousands of tiny receptors of sound), the vestibular system (balance system), and the eighth cranial nerve or acoustic nerve.

Intelligibility: The ability to detect differences among speech sounds, e.g., to hear words such as *manner*, *matter*, and *master* as separate words.

Intensity: Also called loudness, and measured in dB along the side of an audiogram.

Internship: An extended field experience normally carried out under the direction of a training institution and scheduled as the culminating part of a professional training program. The purpose of the internship is to provide the trainee with on-the-job training under the supervision of an experienced practitioner and/or a university supervisor.

Intonation: Variations in pitch patterns (melody) and stress within an utterance (sentence), which add meaning to the message.

Inverse Square Law: The intensity or loudness of a sound decreases 6 dB as the distance between the sound and the receiver is doubled.

Language: A structured symbolic system used to communicate ideas in the form of words, with rules for combining and sequencing these words into thoughts, experiences, or feelings. The language system is comprised of a sound system, a vocabulary or concept system, a word ordering and grammar system and rules for effectively using this symbolic system.

Mainstreaming: The process which promotes integration of the child with a disability to the maximum extent possible in accordance with Federal Public Law 94-142. Integration with "normal" children ranges from full-time placement to integration in classes such as music, art, or gym.

Masking: A procedure often used in hearing testing where a static sound is presented to the nontest ear through the headphones for the purpose of keeping the nontest ear from responding.

Maximum Power Output (MPO, Saturation Sound Pressure Level): The hearing aid has a maximum output limit which cannot be exceeded regardless of how far the gain control is rotated or how high the input sound level becomes. This limitation is a safety factor to prevent uncomfortably loud or harmful sounds.

Middle Ear: That part of the ear comprised of the eardrum, a small air-filled space, and the three smallest bones in the body, all of which function to efficiently conduct sound into the inner ear.

Mixed Hearing Loss: A hearing loss caused by several diseases (pathologies) or problems occurring in different parts of the ear at the same time; can be thought of as having two hearing losses at once, usually conductive and sensorineural.

Office of Handicapped Student Services: The office located in a federally funded college or university that assists in directing and planning a successful course of study for the student with a disability who is attending an institution of higher education.

Open Enrollment: A policy for admitting students to colleges and universities regardless of their academic record. This is also a nonselective admissions process that makes higher education available to more students, usually by accepting any applicant with a high-school diploma.

Otitis Media: Also known as middle-ear infection, the most common cause of conductive hearing loss.

Otologist: Also known as Ear-Nose-Throat (ENT) specialist; a physician who specializes in diseases of the ear.

Outer Ear: That part of the auditory mechanism comprised of the pinna and external auditory meatus (ear canal), which functions to protect and to channel sounds into the middle ear.

Peer Collaboration: Working with one or more other students on learning tasks. This can be especially helpful for clarifying meaning in writing and reading assignments.

Peer Tutoring: Tutoring in particular courses done by students who have done well in those courses. Usually peer tutors also undergo some training in tutoring techniques.

Perception: Occurs in the brainstem and brain and involves learning the meaning of incoming sounds.

Peripheral Mechanism: The outer, middle, and inner ear. Sound is "received" here.

Phonetic Symbols: Markings used to represent the sounds used in a verbal language system.

Post-Secondary Education: Any education obtained following the program received in the public or private sector; beyond high school.

Prerequisite: A requirement, such as completing an elementary course, which must be satisfied before admittance to advanced work.

"Process" Approach: An approach to teaching writing to students that focuses on the stages that a writer may go through in creating a composition, such as prewriting, drafting, revising, and final drafting/editing. The strategy is one of "how to write" and is thus more explanatory in nature than traditional approaches.

"Product" Approach: The traditional method of assigning writing to students. The instructor tells the student what the end product is to be (e.g., descriptive, expository, compare/contrast, etc.); however, no instruction is offered as to the techniques to be employed by the student while they are involved in writing.

Pure Tone: A tone which has energy at only one frequency. These sounds are useful for testing hearing sensitivity because they permit measurement of the contour or configuration of the hearing loss.

Pure Tone Air Conduction Testing: That part of a basic hearing test battery where whistle-like sounds are presented to each ear separately through headphones, and the individual raises his/her hand each time he/she can just barely hear the tone.

Pure Tone Bone Conduction Testing: That part of a basic hearing test battery where whistle-like sounds are presented through a bone-oscillator, and the individual raises his/her hand each time he/she can just barely hear the tone.

Reception: The actual detection of the sound which occurs in the inner ear.

Receptive Language: Skills involving the ability to receive and comprehend the language that one hears in the environment.

Residual Hearing: The hearing that remains when one has a hearing loss. There is almost always some residual or remaining hearing, even with the most profound hearing losses.

Résumé: A brief, written summary including biographical information, educational background, and work history.

Reverberation: The amount of echo in a room.

SAT: The Scholastic Aptitude Test (SAT) is a test developed by the Educational Testing Service for the College Entrance Examination Board. It is to be used for college-admission decisions and college counseling.

Secondary Language: Skills that involve higher level language such as reading and writing as opposed to listening and speaking.

Sensorineural Hearing Loss: A hearing loss (also called a nerve loss) which occurs when the pathology is located in the inner ear or auditory nerve. It is usually a permanent hearing loss.

Sensorineural Mechanism: That part of the entire ear structure which includes the inner ear and acoustic nerve.

SHHH: Means "Self Help for Hard-of-Hearing People"; a consumer oriented journal and group with national and local chapters.

Signal-to-Noise Ratio: The relationship between the signal of choice and anything else that the person does not want to hear. A person with a hearing loss needs the signal to be about ten times louder than background sounds.

Site of Lesion: The place in the auditory system where the disease or damage occurs that is causing the hearing loss (e.g., middle ear or inner ear). A good hearing test reveals site of lesion.

Sound Field Testing: The process in which some aspect of hearing is tested by sounds that come from a loudspeaker as opposed to earphones.

Speech-Language Pathologist: A certified individual with a graduate degree who specializes in the assessment and treatment of communication disorders.

Speech Reception or Recognition Threshold (SRT): The specific test in the basic hearing test battery which finds the softest level at which an individual can just barely understand speech fifty percent of the time.

Speech Sound Improvement: Therapy directed at improving the production of specific sounds such as "r, s, l, sh, ch," etc.

Support Services: Ancillary services that are provided to assist a child in achieving academic success such as speech- language therapy, aural habilitation, tutoring, etc.

Telecoil Switch: The control on a hearing aid that turns off the microphone and activates a telecoil in the aid which picks up magnetic leakage from a telephone, or a loop of an ALD.

Threshold: That point where the individual can just barely hear a sound fifty percent of the time. All sounds louder than threshold can be heard, sounds softer cannot be detected.

Tinnitus: Also called "ringing in the ears." Any of a number of internal head sounds which often accompany a hearing loss.

Trouble Shooting (hearing aids): Performing various auditory and visual inspections when a hearing aid malfunctions in order to determine the nature and severity of the problem.

Tuning Fork Tests: Part of a basic hearing test battery which involves a quick, subjective screen of type and degree of hearing loss, at the frequency (pitch) of the fork.

Two-year Program: The two-year program offers two years of college-level work. The student follows an organized curriculum leading to a formal award, such as an associate degree.

University Speech and Hearing Clinic: A speech and hearing facility which is part of a university and functions as a laboratory to train students, as well as to provide services to the university and community.

Vent (of an earmold): A second hole or opening through the earmold in addition to the opening for sound from the hearing aid. Traditionally, vents have been used to reduce low-frequency amplification for individuals who have good hearing sensitivity for low pitched sounds.

Vestibular System: Located in the inner ear and has to do with regulating balance.

Vocational Education: A secondary or adult educational program aimed at preparation of specific occupational skills and general work behaviors leading to paid employment.

Vocational Rehabilitation Counselor: A professional who assists persons with disabilities in the development of an individualized plan leading to employment and to a career.

Word Discrimination Testing: Also called word identification testing. Part of a basic hearing test battery, where one determines how well words can be discriminated when they are presented at a typical conversational-level of loudness, and at an additional level loud enough to overcome the individual's hearing loss.

NOTES

NOTES